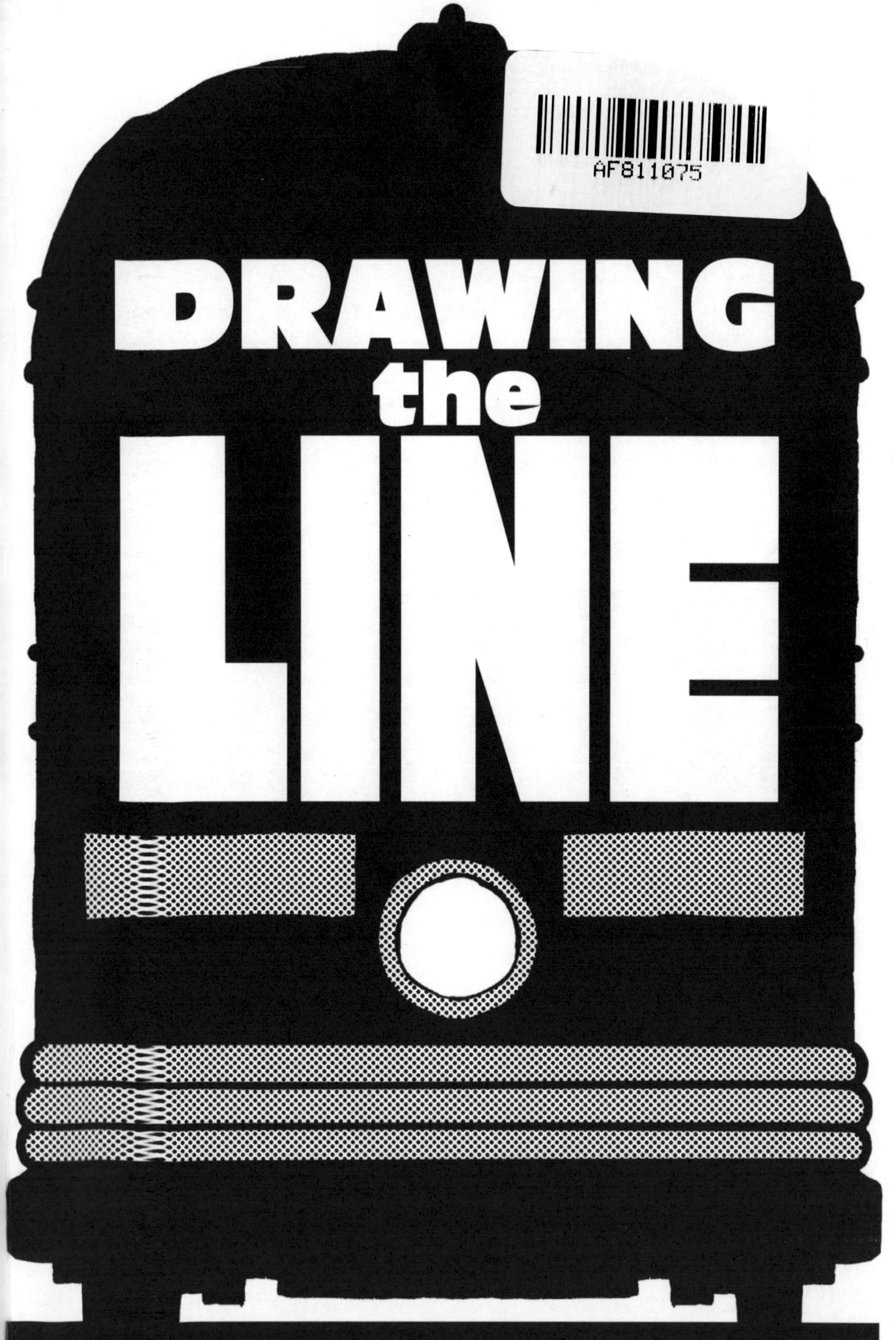
DRAWING
the
LINE

DRAWING THE LINE - May 2004

First Edition: May 2004
ISBN: 0-9735116-0-3

Printed in Canada

Book layout and design by Ron Boyd

How Drawing The Line came to be ...

by Suley

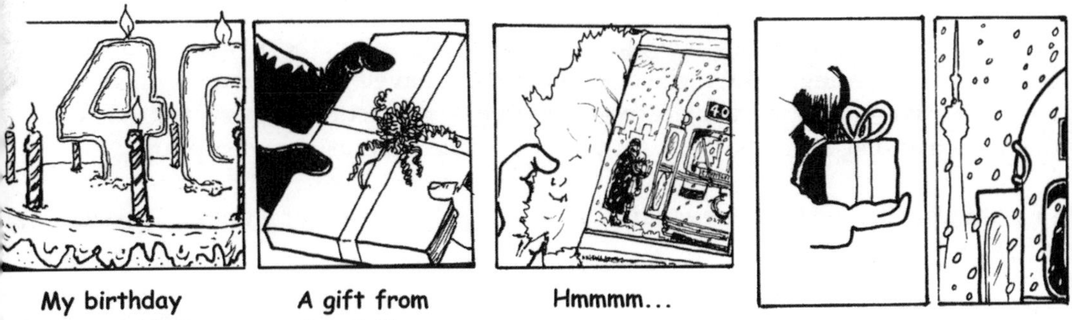

My birthday February 2003. | A gift from Ron & Kim. | Hmmmm...

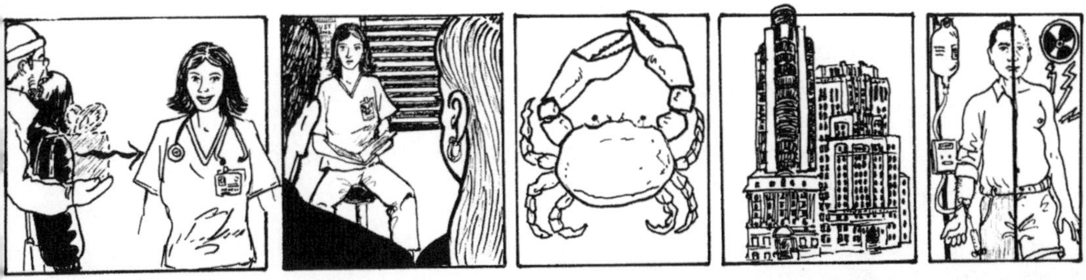

Kim is both friend and doctor. | August 2002. | Diagnosis: CANCER (It's curable) | I was treated here, at PMH. | Both chemo and radiation.

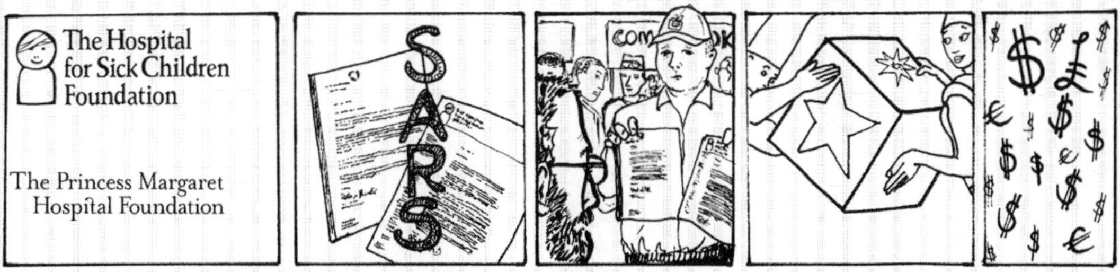

March 2003: IDEA! A benefit comic book. | Endoresments; then SARS hits. | Artists are inspired and participate. | Their contributions come in ... | ... as do private donations!

This book is the result.

All proceeds from the sale of this book, benefiting cancer research, will be shared equally between The Hospital for Sick Children Foundation and Princess Margaret Hospital Foundation.

The art and stories in Drawing The Line are ideas and views by the artists and not those of The Hospital for Sick Children nor Princess Margaret Hospital. Although children may read this book, this book is not intended for children.

With thanks...

This book is the product of 15 months worth of work. From the artwork and stories, to editing, to printing, to financial donations, there have been so many selfless people who have stepped up to the plate to aid me in the production of this comic book. I thank each and every one of you, for your patience, generosity and support.

I would also like to acknowledge the following people, without whom this book would not exist:

All the artists, particularly RG Taylor and Mark Askwith who both are invaluable resources. My advisors: Stephanie Hunter; Peter Birkemoe and Chris Butcher; Peter & Irene Dixon, Kevin Boyd and Doug Simpson.

All our donors who believed in this project and participated wholeheartedly, without hesitation, and with amazing generosity.

Sofia Ramirez and Wendy Howze of the hospital foundations for moving mountains and finding solutions.

To Ron and Kim, my deepest thanks for sparking the idea and being there from day one.

A special thank you to my parents for all their unconditional love and support.

The greatest of thanks must go to Julie Eng who was there through thick and thin and who is the backbone of this project. The website, the exhibit at the Frecklebean Café and the book would not exist without her tireless creativity, her effervescence and her love.

I can never thank you enough.

Suley

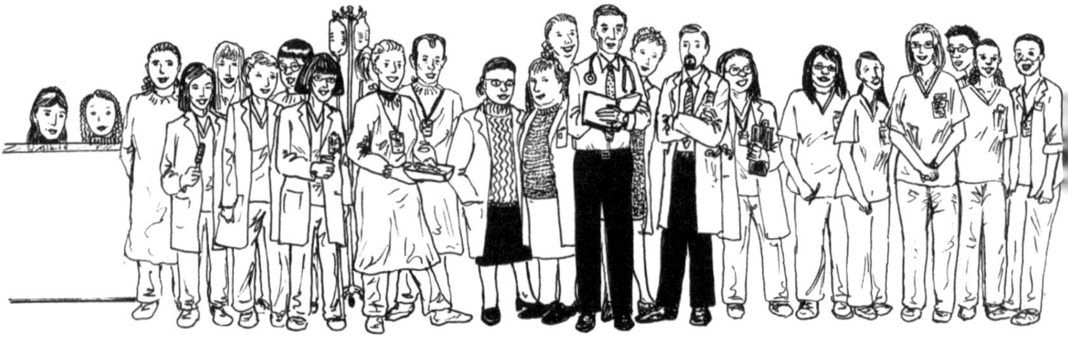

This book is dedicated to all the doctors, nurses, technicians and administrative staff, in particular those who have enriched my experience and eased my journey.

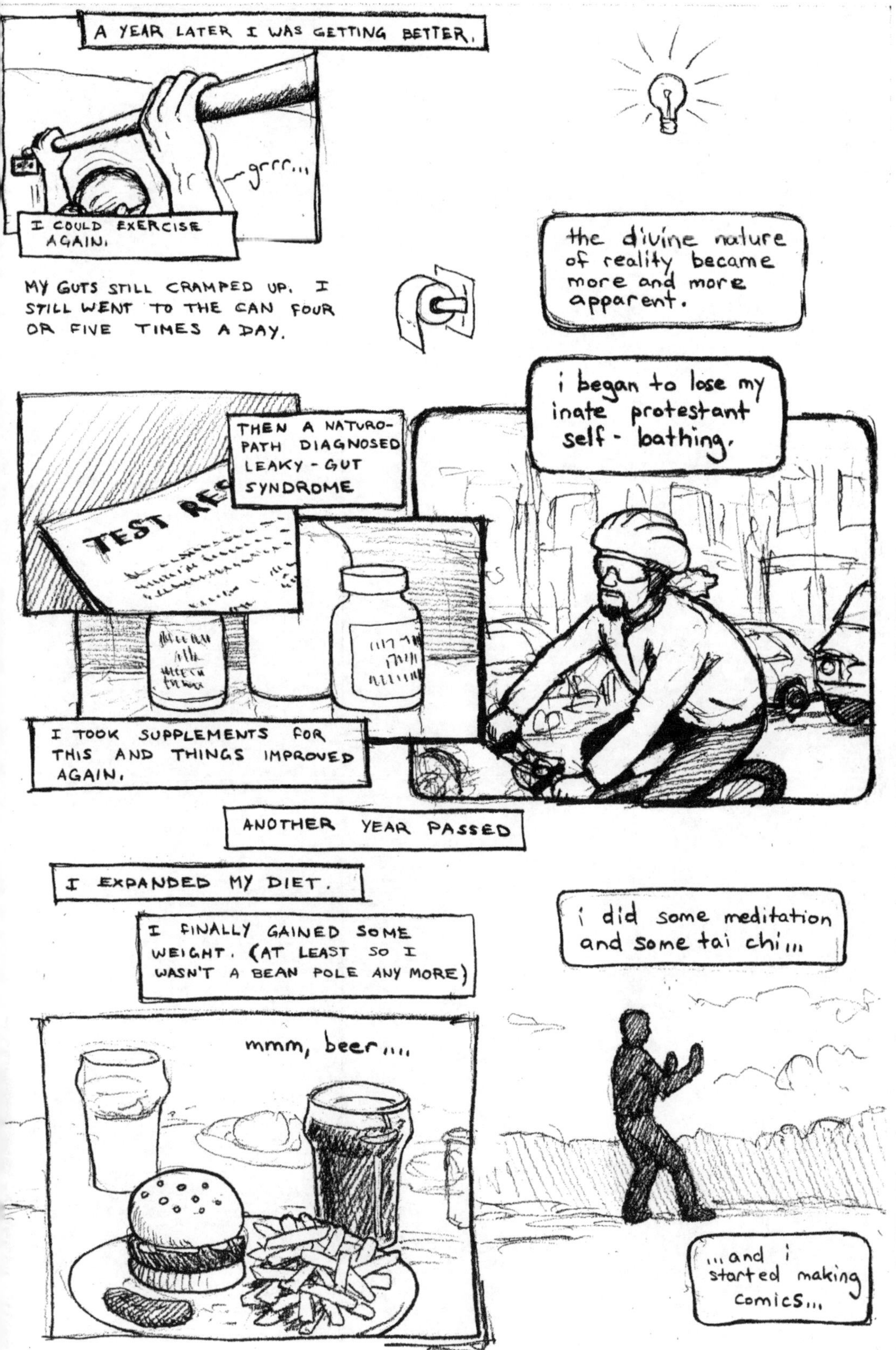
A YEAR LATER I WAS GETTING BETTER.
~grrr...
I COULD EXERCISE AGAIN.
MY GUTS STILL CRAMPED UP. I STILL WENT TO THE CAN FOUR OR FIVE TIMES A DAY.
the divine nature of reality became more and more apparent.
THEN A NATURO-PATH DIAGNOSED LEAKY-GUT SYNDROME
TEST RES
i began to lose my inate protestant self-bathing.
I TOOK SUPPLEMENTS FOR THIS AND THINGS IMPROVED AGAIN.
ANOTHER YEAR PASSED
I EXPANDED MY DIET.
I FINALLY GAINED SOME WEIGHT. (AT LEAST SO I WASN'T A BEAN POLE ANY MORE)
i did some meditation and some tai chi...
mmm, beer....
...and i started making comics...

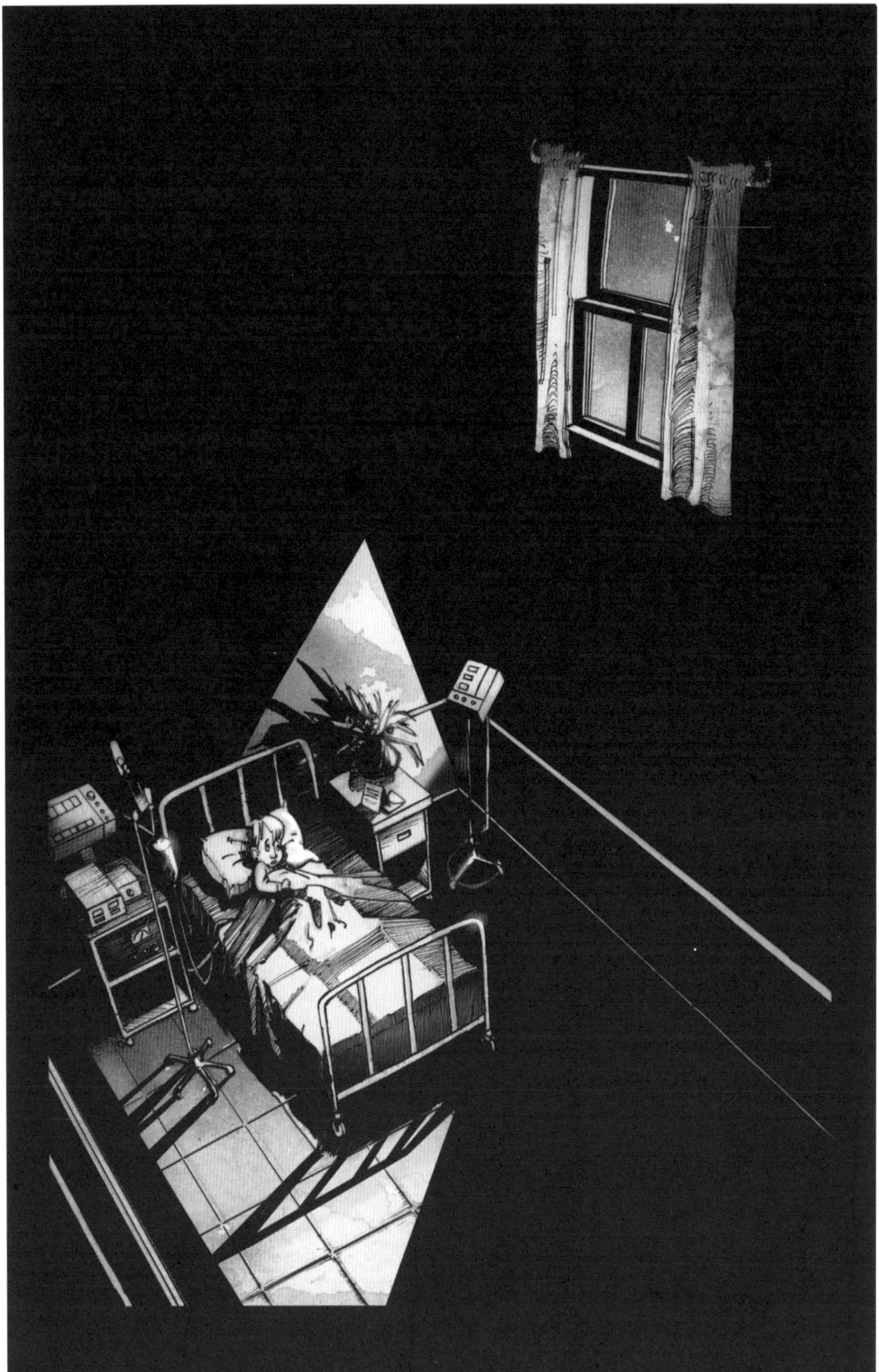

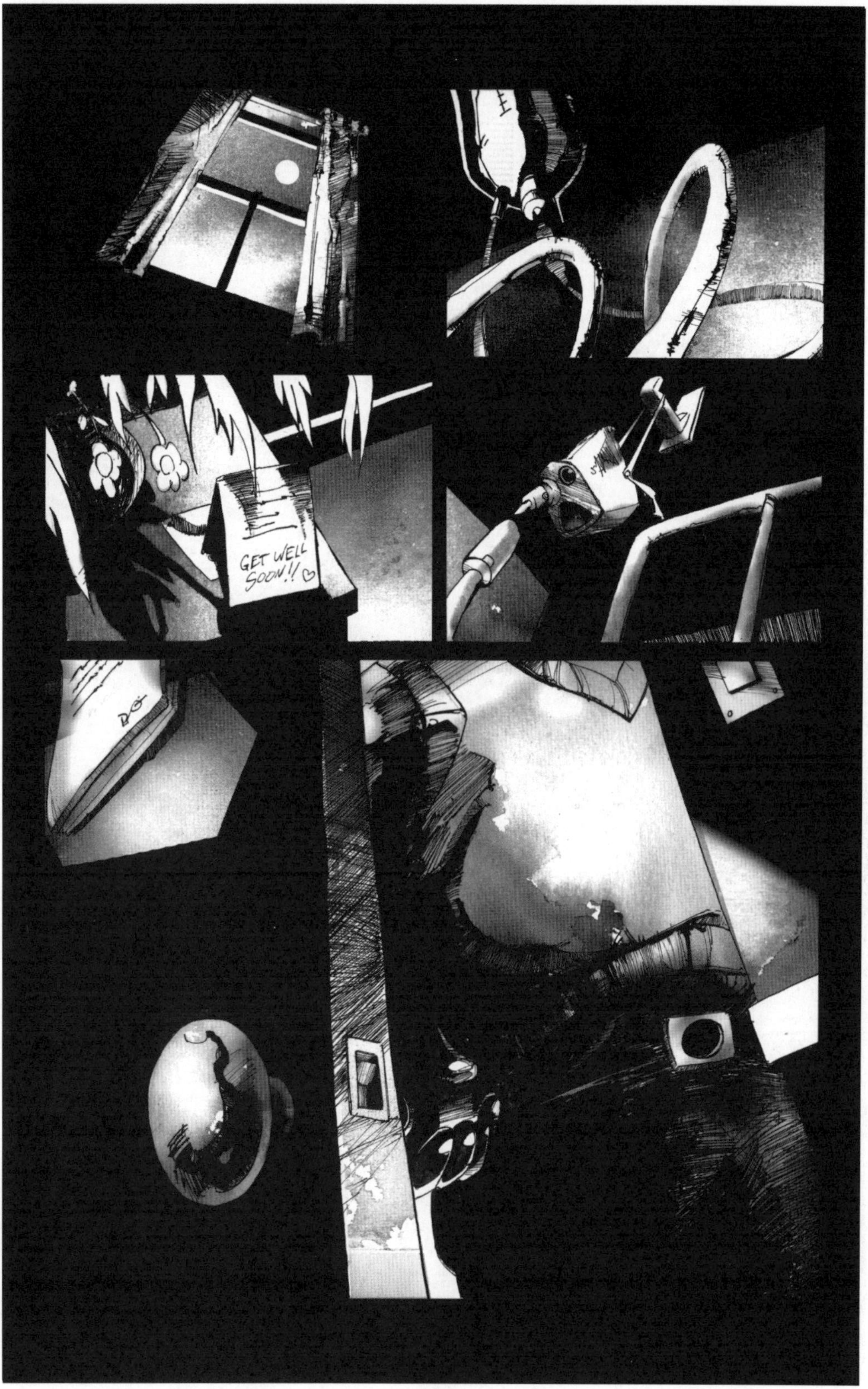
GET WELL
SOON!! ♡

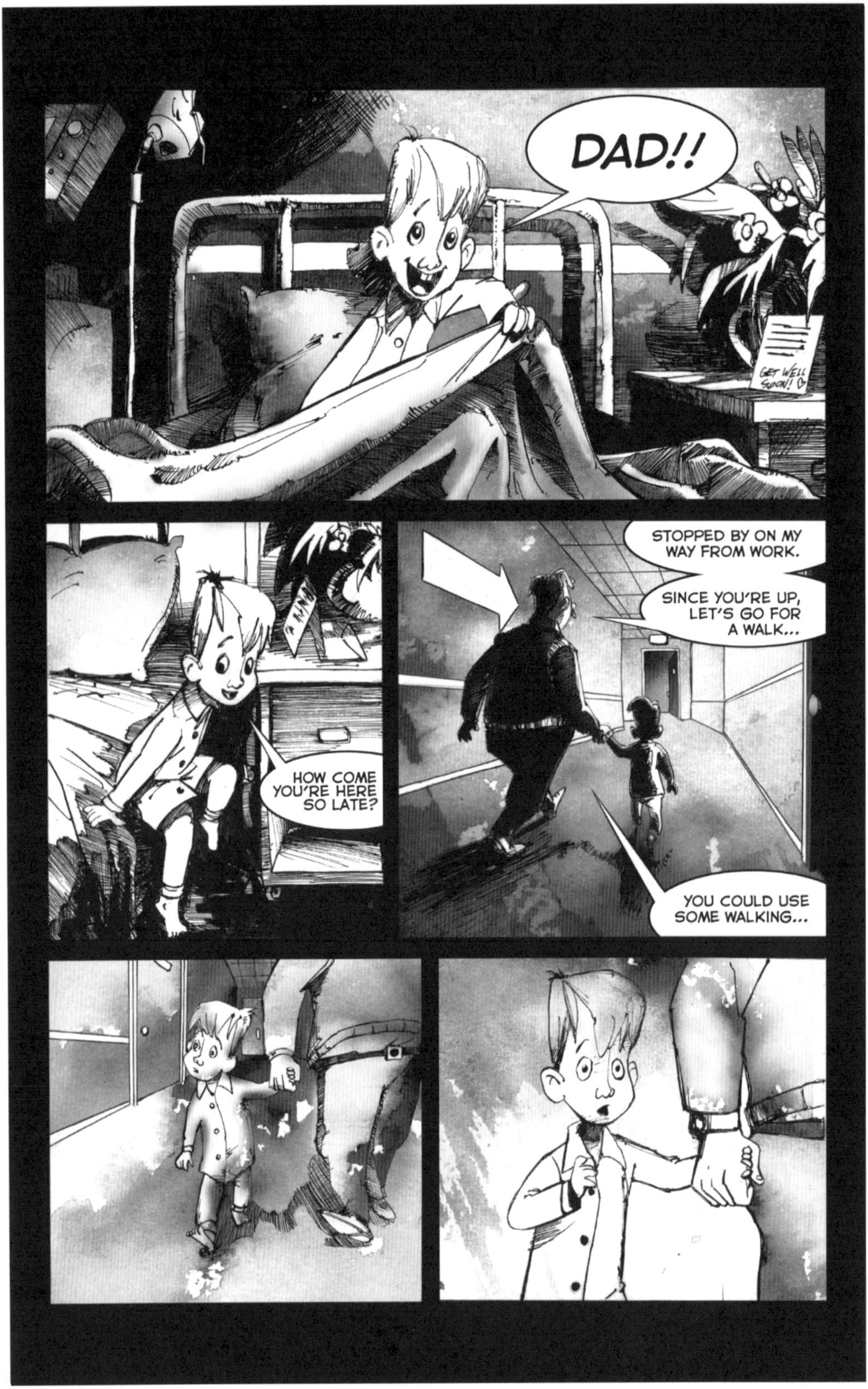
DAD!!
GET WELL SOON!
HOW COME YOU'RE HERE SO LATE?
STOPPED BY ON MY WAY FROM WORK.
SINCE YOU'RE UP, LET'S GO FOR A WALK...
YOU COULD USE SOME WALKING...

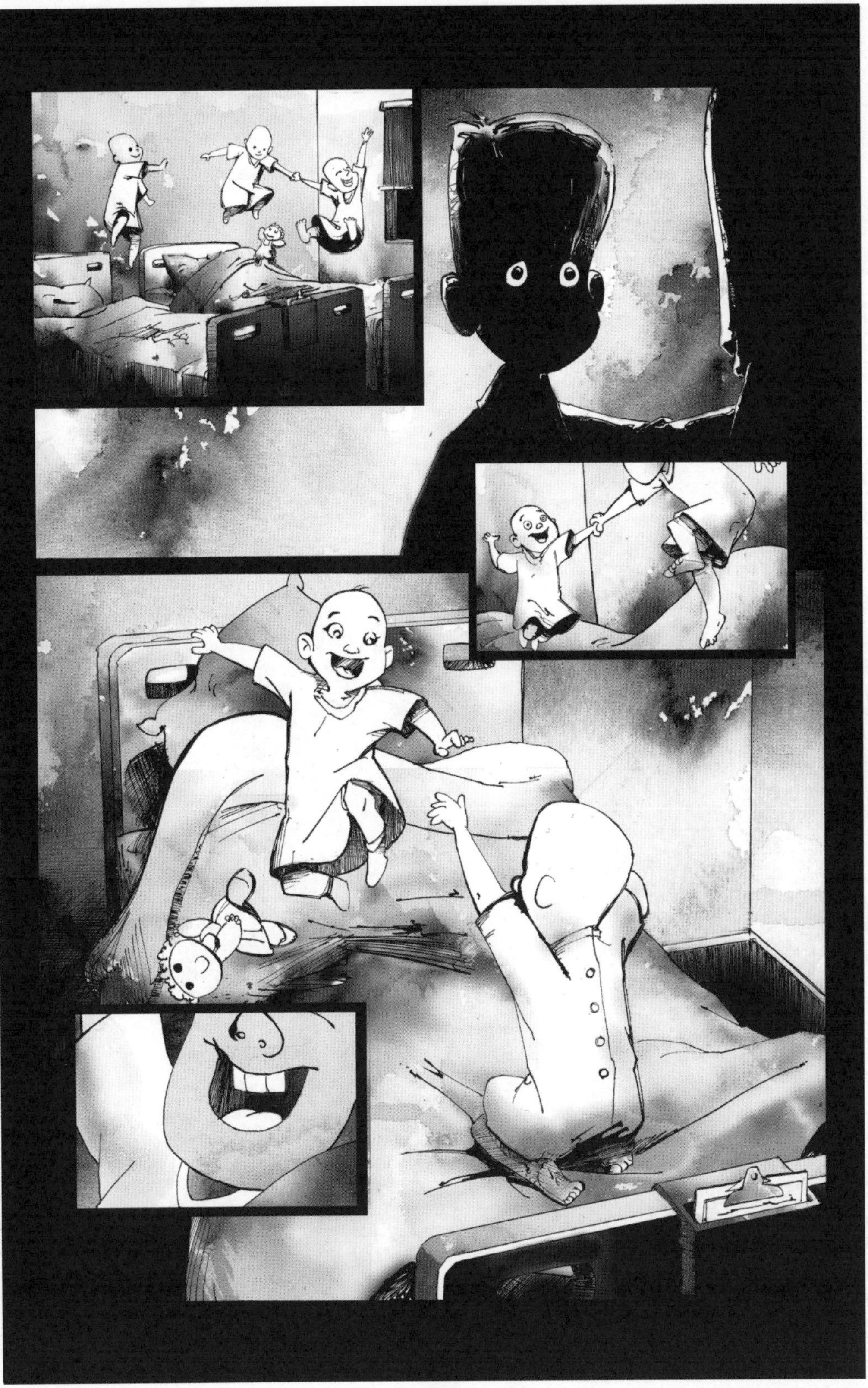

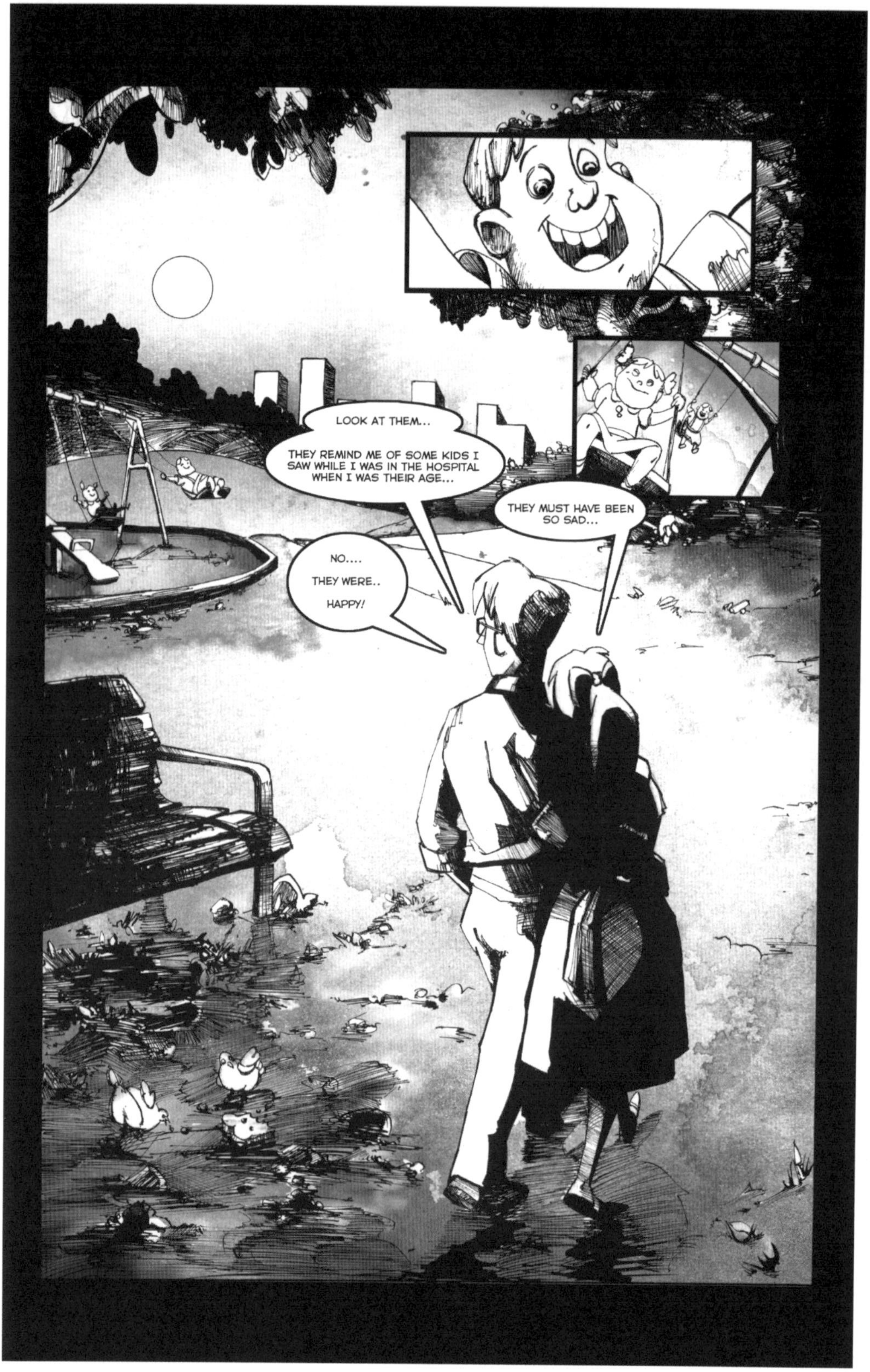
LOOK AT THEM...
THEY REMIND ME OF SOME KIDS I SAW WHILE I WAS IN THE HOSPITAL WHEN I WAS THEIR AGE...
THEY MUST HAVE BEEN SO SAD...
NO.... THEY WERE.. HAPPY!

This is the story of...

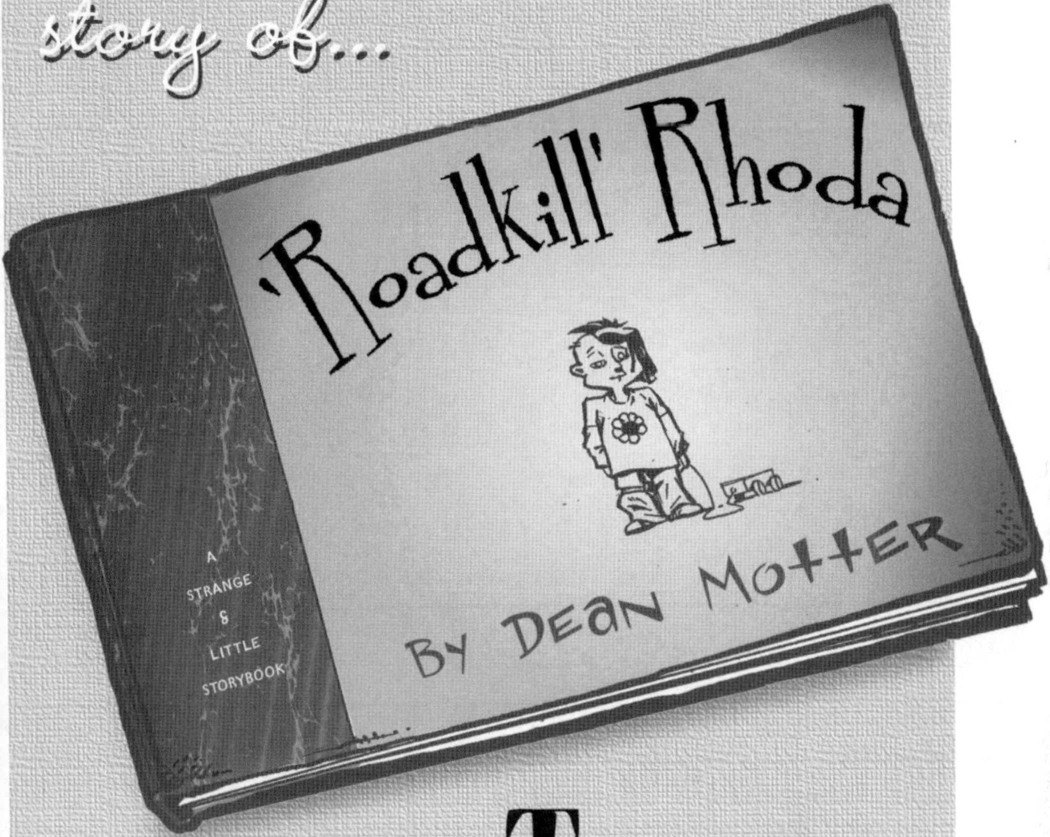

There once was a little girl named Rhoda. One day while playing in the street she was run over by an S.U.V. driven by a soccer mom talking on her cell-phone.

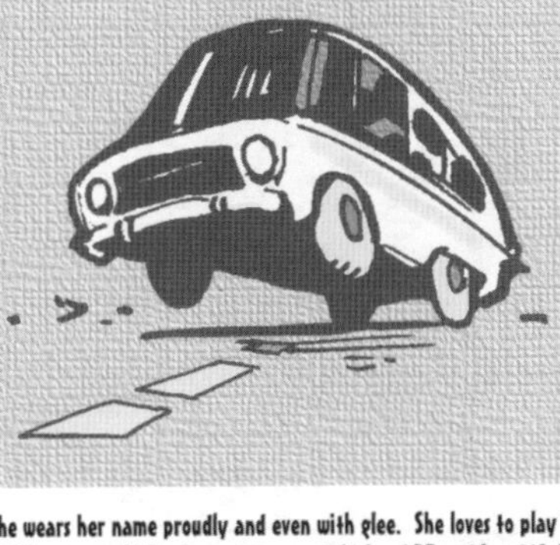

For the real-life 'Roadkill' whom I met in Ward C. She wears her name proudly and even with glee. She loves to play 'Go Fish' and excels at 'Red Rover.'
Her playmates all tremble when they hear, "Let Roadkill come over!" She loves eating sandwhichs of PB and J and if they would let her would eat them all day.
At eight years of age she has been through a lot. She has been through some things that she would rather have not.
I am lucky to know her-- and don't think I'm nuts: though some may be missing, I admire her guts. - *To Rhoda From Dean*

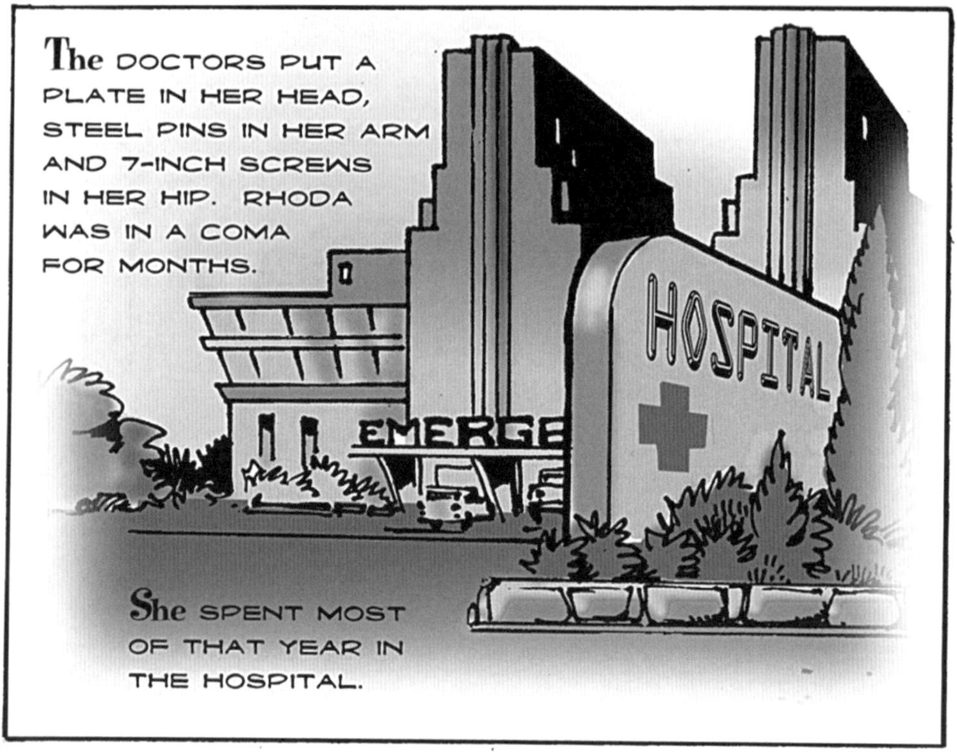
The DOCTORS PUT A PLATE IN HER HEAD, STEEL PINS IN HER ARM AND 7-INCH SCREWS IN HER HIP. RHODA WAS IN A COMA FOR MONTHS.
HOSPITAL
EMERGE
She SPENT MOST OF THAT YEAR IN THE HOSPITAL.

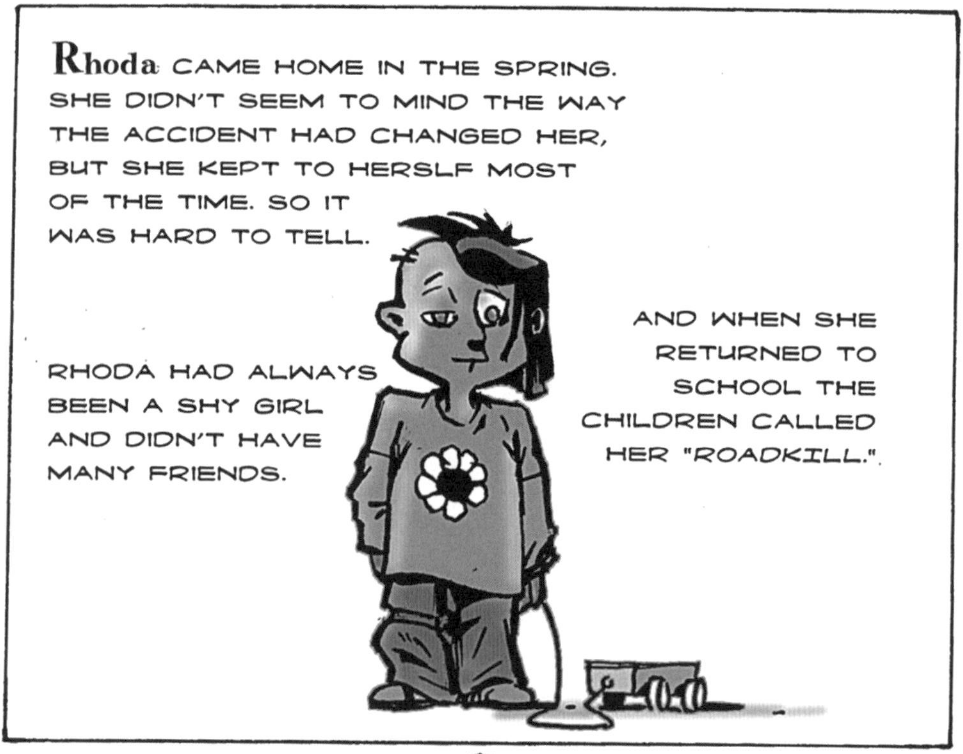
Rhoda CAME HOME IN THE SPRING. SHE DIDN'T SEEM TO MIND THE WAY THE ACCIDENT HAD CHANGED HER, BUT SHE KEPT TO HERSLF MOST OF THE TIME. SO IT WAS HARD TO TELL.
RHODA HAD ALWAYS BEEN A SHY GIRL AND DIDN'T HAVE MANY FRIENDS.
AND WHEN SHE RETURNED TO SCHOOL THE CHILDREN CALLED HER "ROADKILL."

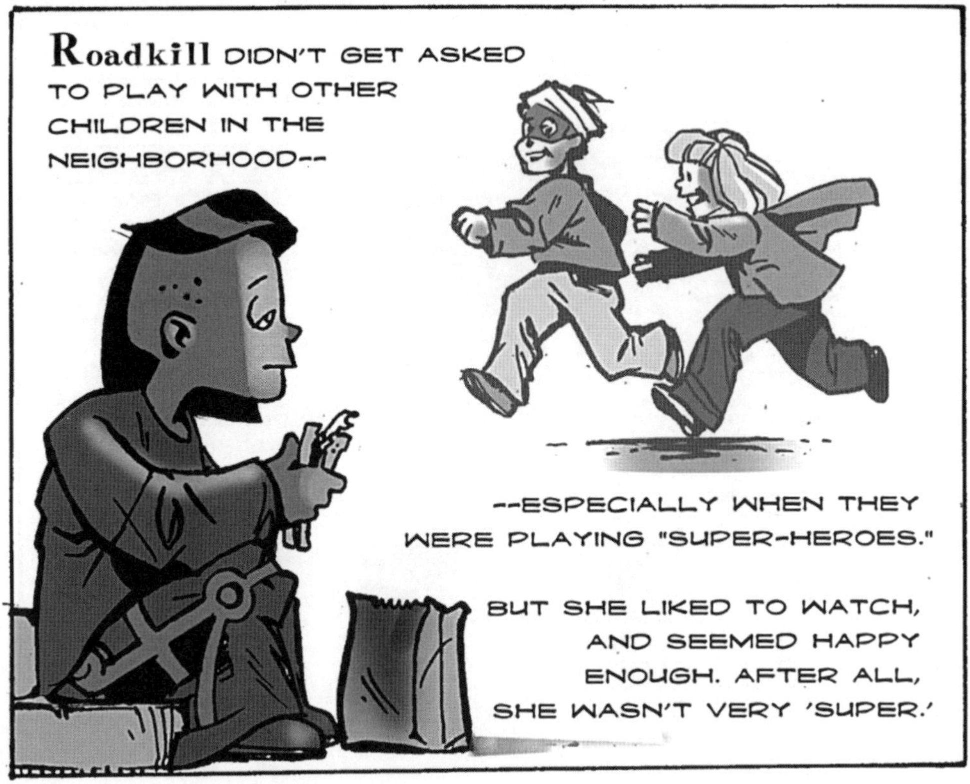
Roadkill DIDN'T GET ASKED TO PLAY WITH OTHER CHILDREN IN THE NEIGHBORHOOD--
--ESPECIALLY WHEN THEY WERE PLAYING "SUPER-HEROES."
BUT SHE LIKED TO WATCH, AND SEEMED HAPPY ENOUGH. AFTER ALL, SHE WASN'T VERY 'SUPER.'

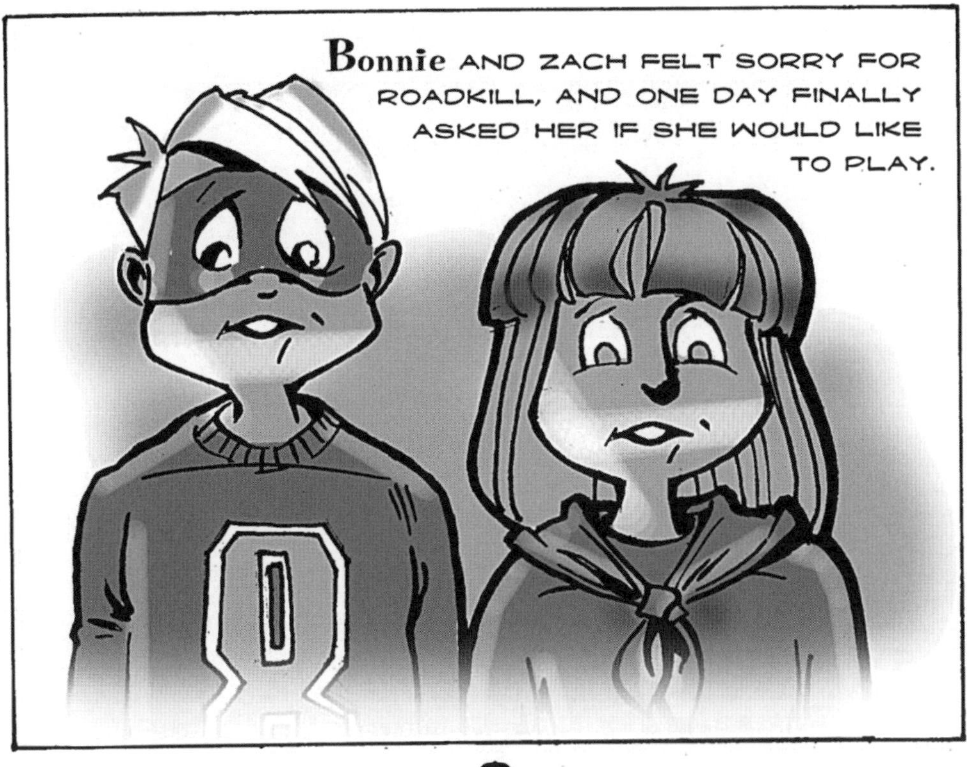
Bonnie AND ZACH FELT SORRY FOR ROADKILL, AND ONE DAY FINALLY ASKED HER IF SHE WOULD LIKE TO PLAY.

"I CAN'T BE SUPER-HUMAN." SAID ROADKILL. "I DON'T HAVE ANY POWERS,"

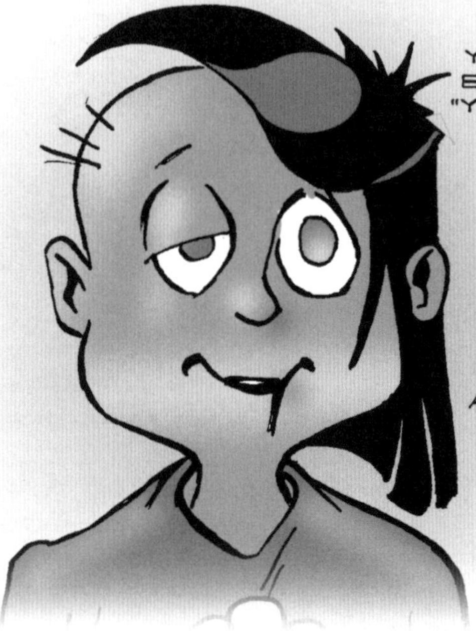

"SURE YOU CAN. YOU'RE A CYBORG!" EXCLAIMED BONNIE. "YOU'RE EVEN *MORE* THAN HUMAN. I WISH WE COULD BE LIKE YOU, *CYBORG.*"

THEN ROADKILL KNEW HOW TO PLAY WITH HER NEW FRIENDS.

"I KNOW! LET'S ALL BE *CYBORGS!*"

"YEAH?" SAID ZACH. "HOW?"

"JUST FOLLOW ME!"

And OFF THE NEW CHUMS WENT TO PLAY.

"BUT NOT ON THE FOUR-LANE HIGHWAY THIS TIME!" SAID ROADKILL.

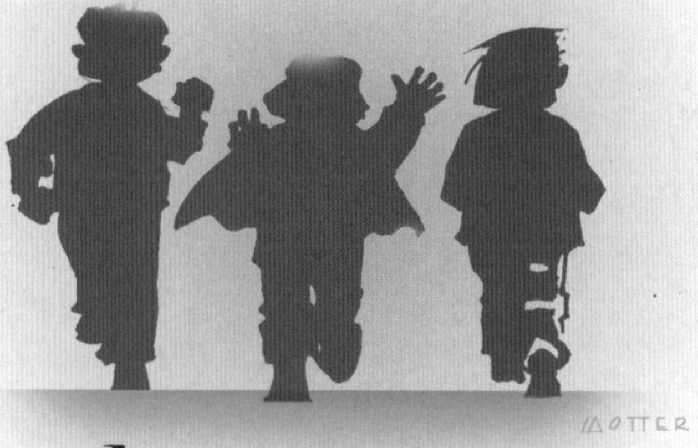

Moral: SUPER-HUMAN OR CYBORG--
IT'S JUST TOO DARN EASY TO END UP AS ROADKILL.

LIVE LIFE. PLAY SAFE. YADDA YADDA.

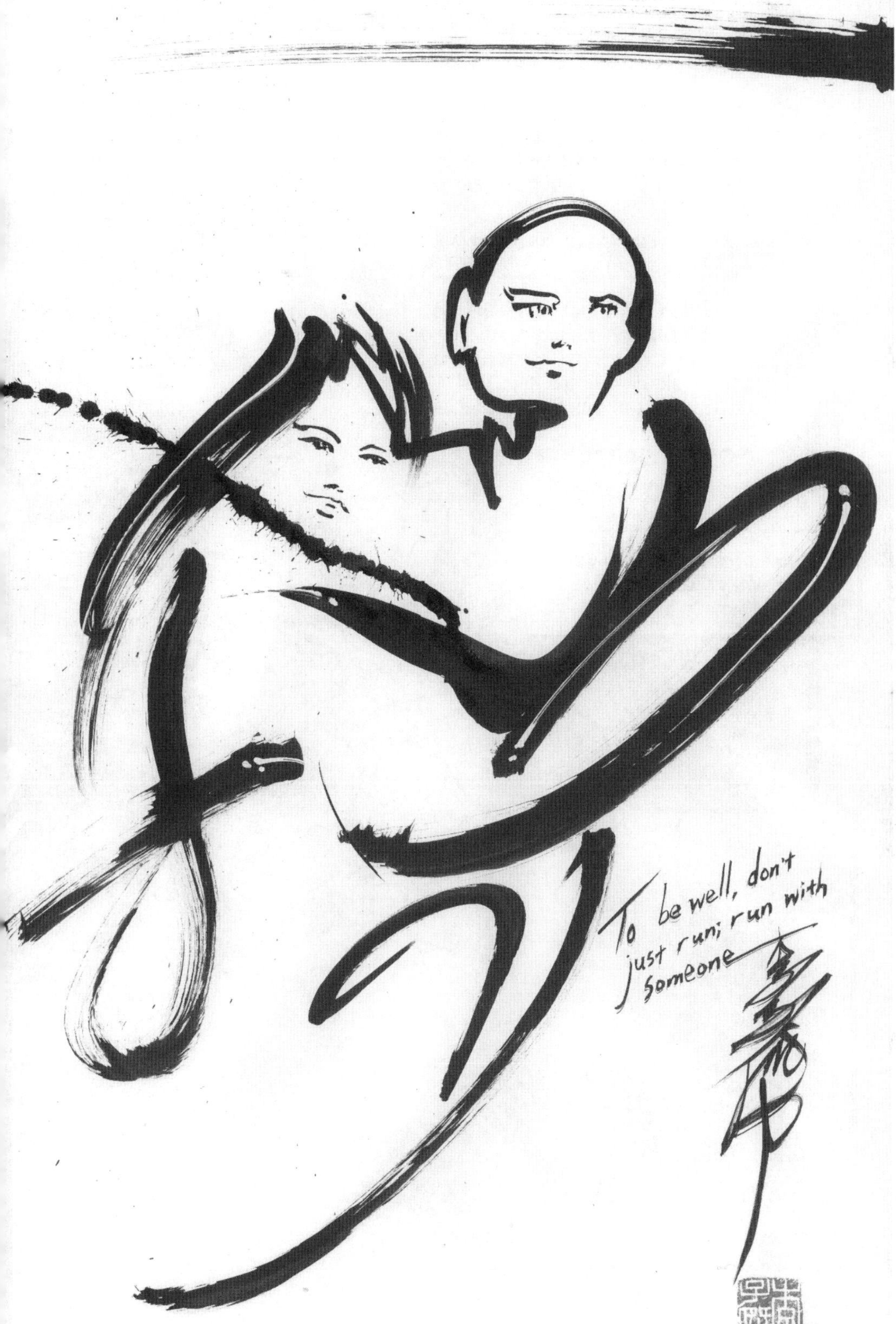
To be well, don't just run; run with someone

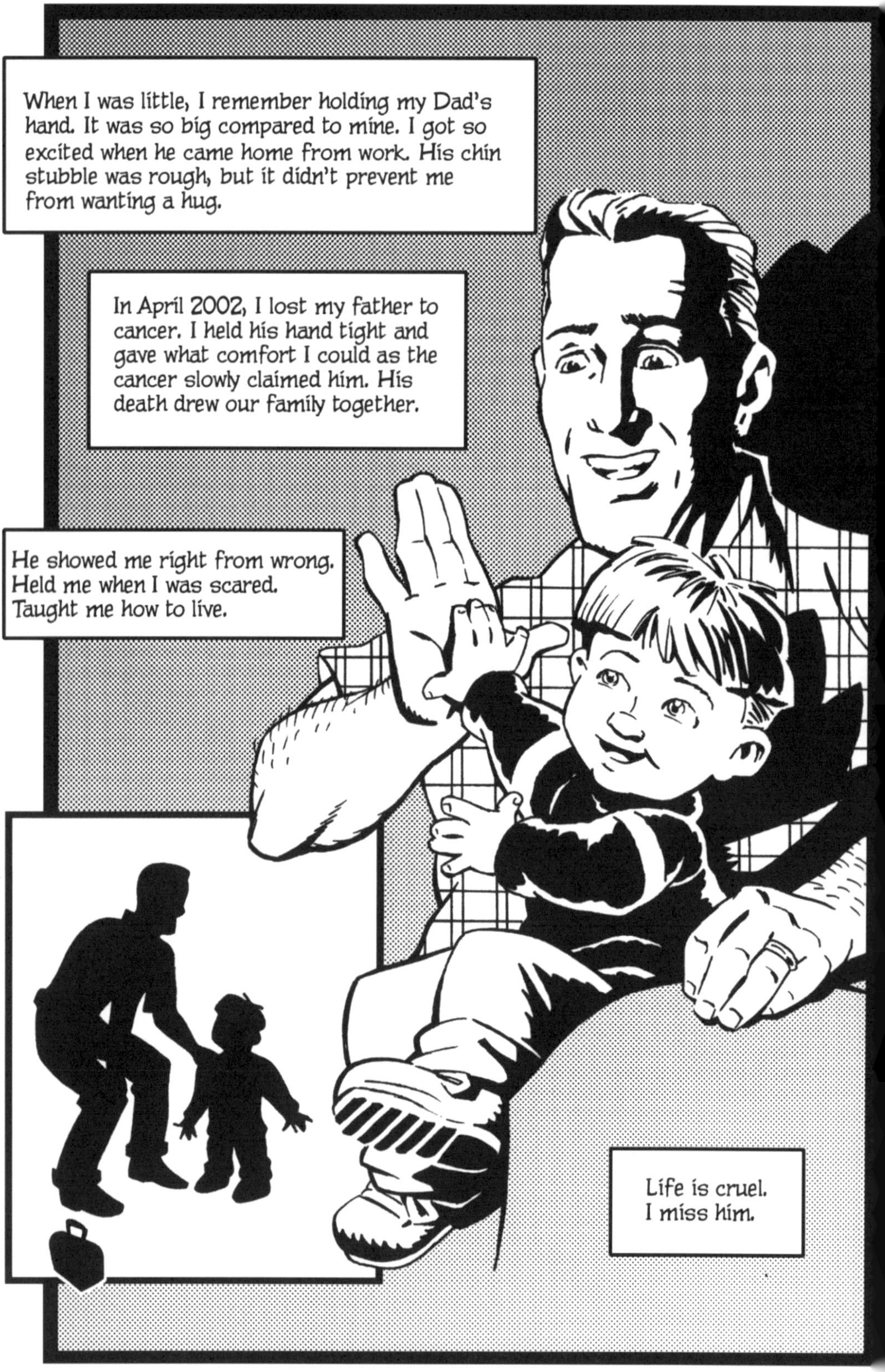
When I was little, I remember holding my Dad's hand. It was so big compared to mine. I got so excited when he came home from work. His chin stubble was rough, but it didn't prevent me from wanting a hug.
In April 2002, I lost my father to cancer. I held his hand tight and gave what comfort I could as the cancer slowly claimed him. His death drew our family together.
He showed me right from wrong. Held me when I was scared. Taught me how to live.
Life is cruel. I miss him.

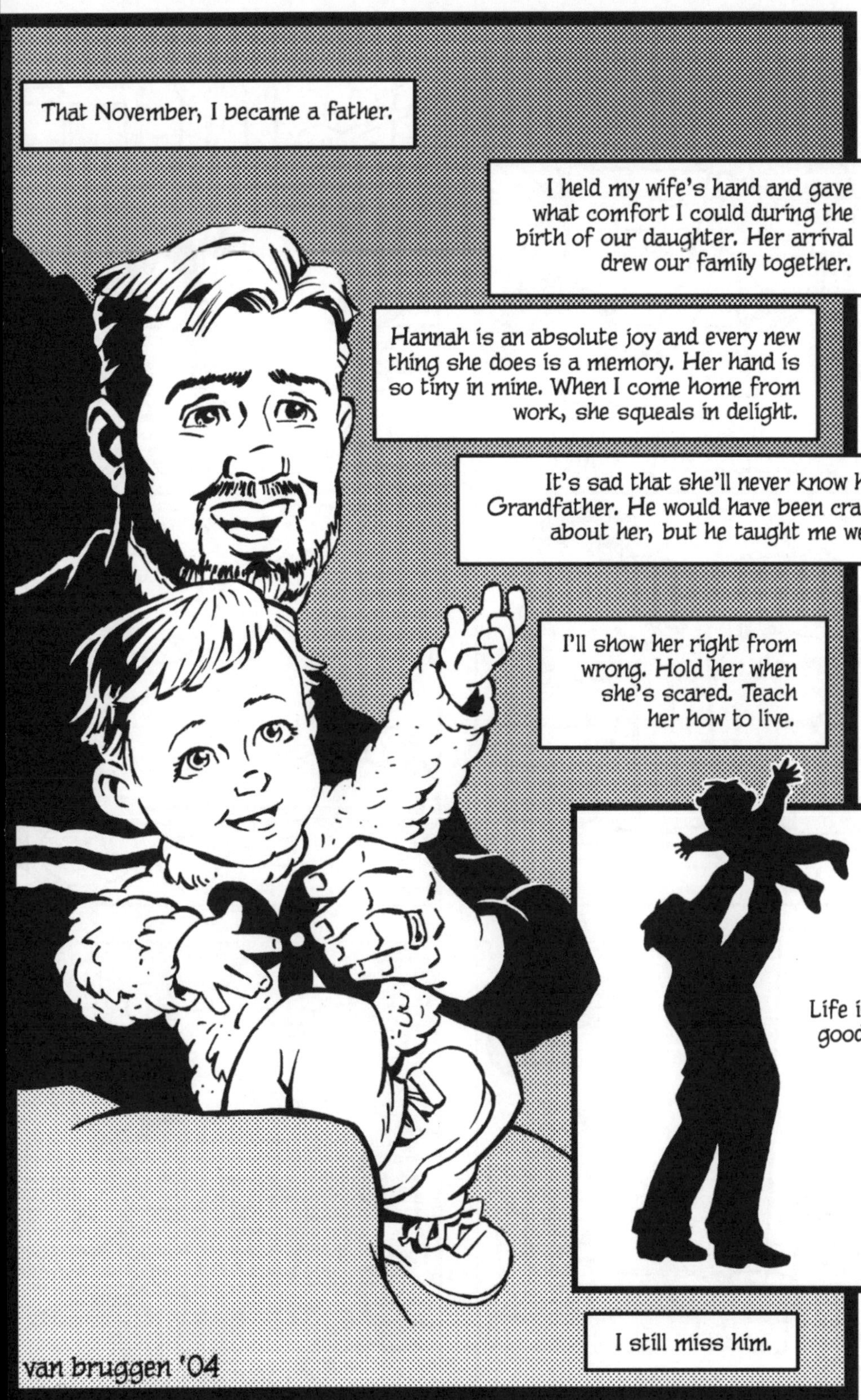
That November, I became a father.
I held my wife's hand and gave what comfort I could during the birth of our daughter. Her arrival drew our family together.
Hannah is an absolute joy and every new thing she does is a memory. Her hand is so tiny in mine. When I come home from work, she squeals in delight.
It's sad that she'll never know her Grandfather. He would have been crazy about her, but he taught me well.
I'll show her right from wrong. Hold her when she's scared. Teach her how to live.
Life is good.
I still miss him.
van bruggen '04

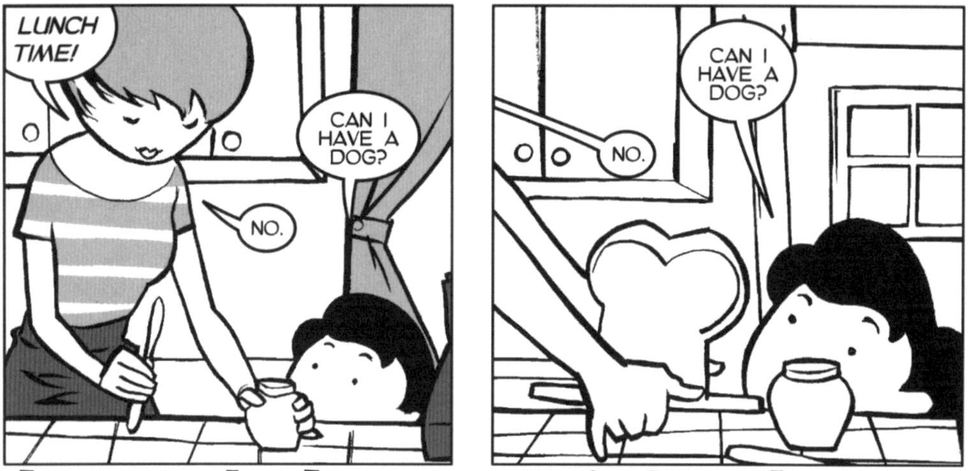

Jeopardy Jones in Fair Trade

story by kathryn kuder & stuart immonen

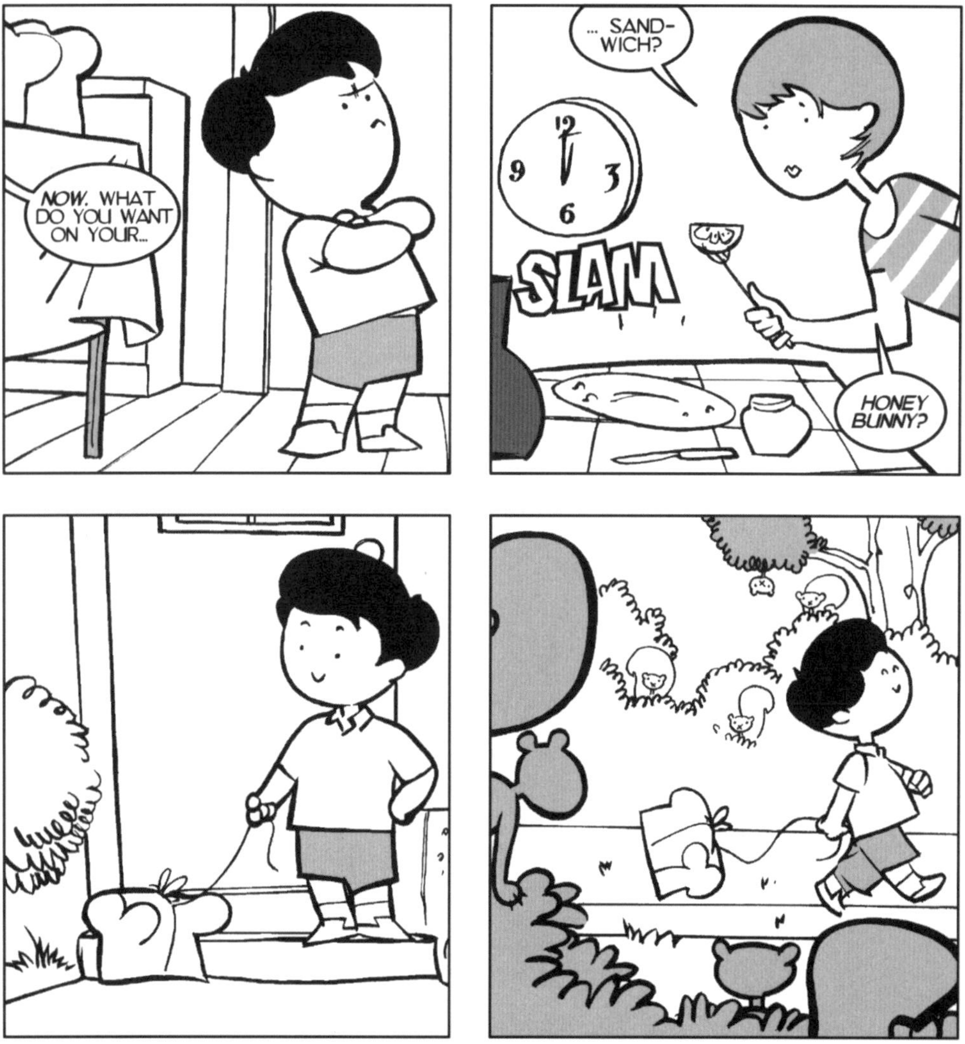

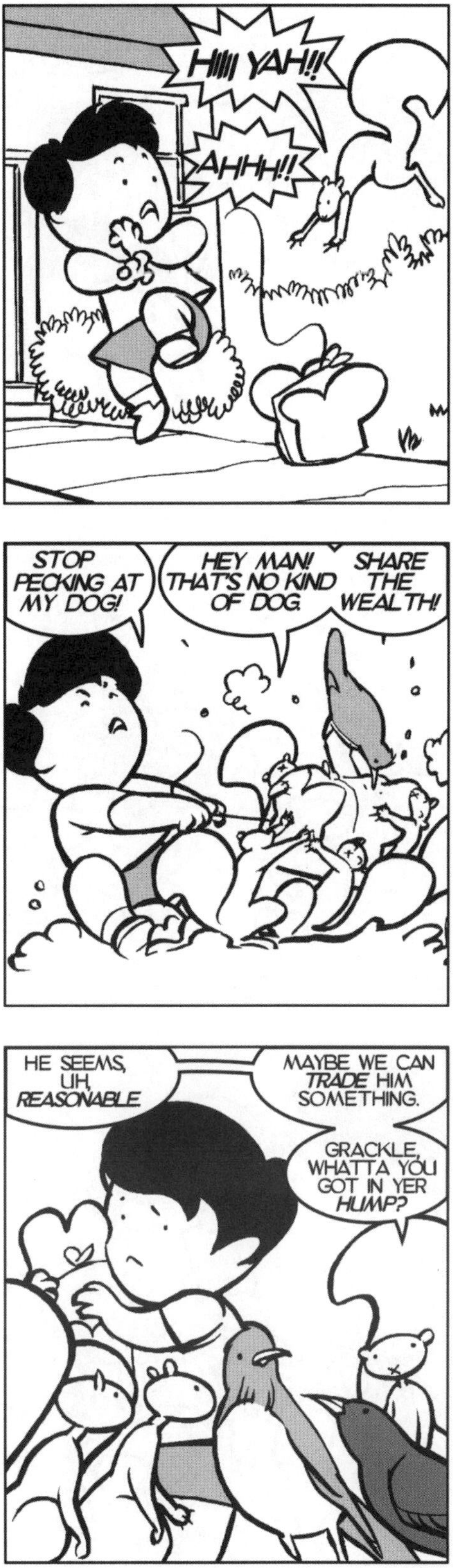
HIIII YAH!!
AHHH!!
I'M A BEAST WITH THE YEAST!
GET OFF MY DOG!
STOP PECKING AT MY DOG!
HEY MAN! THAT'S NO KIND OF DOG.
SHARE THE WEALTH!
NO WAY! IT'S THE KINDA DOG I GOT!
NOW BACK OFF!!
OKAY, OKAY. WE'RE ALL CIVILIZED ANIMALS HERE.
HE SEEMS, UH, REASONABLE.
MAYBE WE CAN TRADE HIM SOMETHING.
GRACKLE, WHATTA YOU GOT IN YER HUMP?
I KNOW IT'S IN HERE SOMEWHERE...
WAAAY BETTER THAN SOME DOG...
AHA!

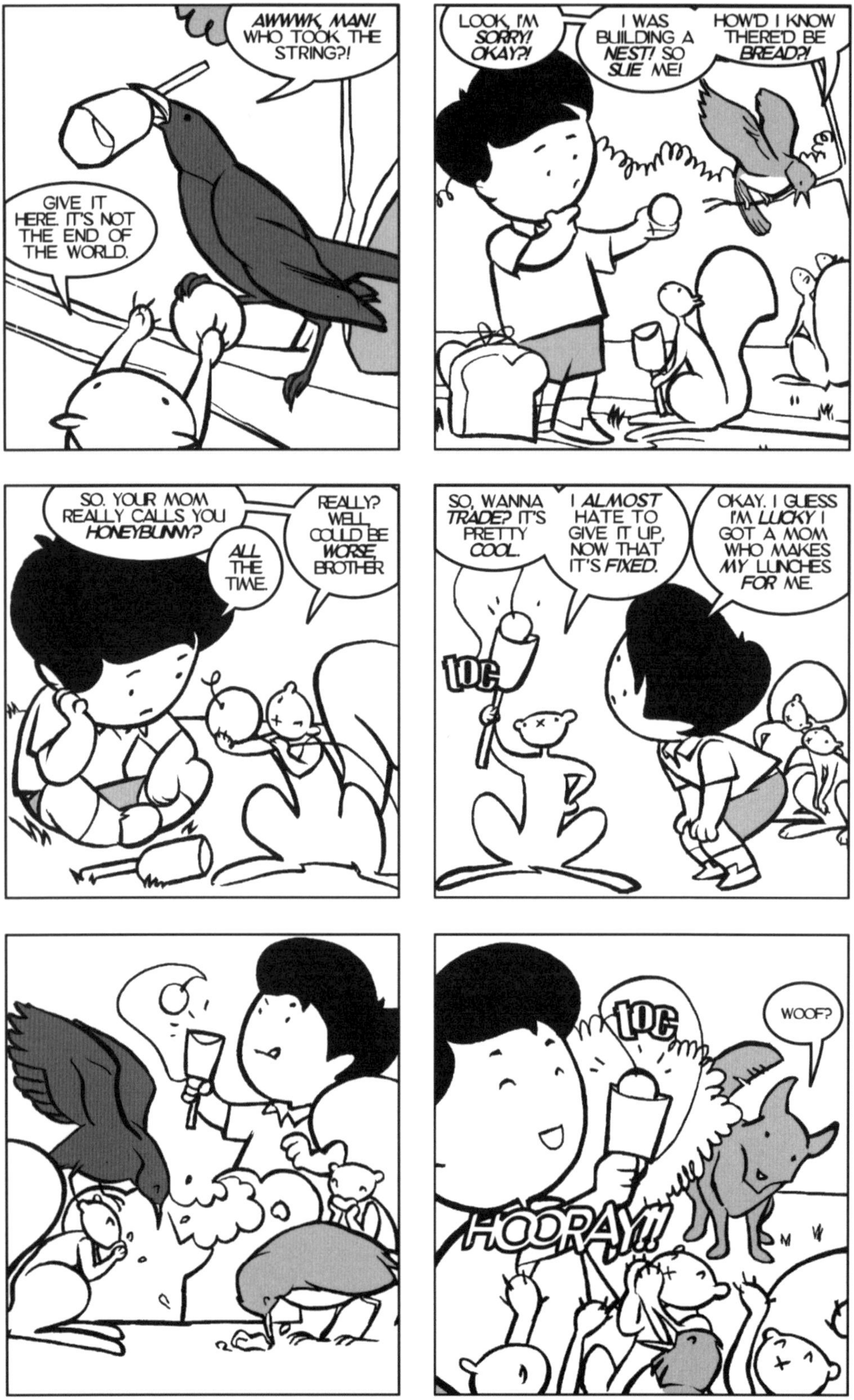
AWWWK, MAN! WHO TOOK THE STRING?!
GIVE IT HERE. IT'S NOT THE END OF THE WORLD.
LOOK, I'M SORRY! OKAY?!
I WAS BUILDING A NEST! SO SUE ME!
HOW'D I KNOW THERE'D BE BREAD?!
SO. YOUR MOM REALLY CALLS YOU HONEYBUNNY?
ALL THE TIME.
REALLY? WELL, COULD BE WORSE, BROTHER.
SO, WANNA TRADE? IT'S PRETTY COOL.
I ALMOST HATE TO GIVE IT UP, NOW THAT IT'S FIXED.
toc
OKAY. I GUESS I'M LUCKY I GOT A MOM WHO MAKES MY LUNCHES FOR ME.
toc
WOOF?
HOORAY!!

Fin

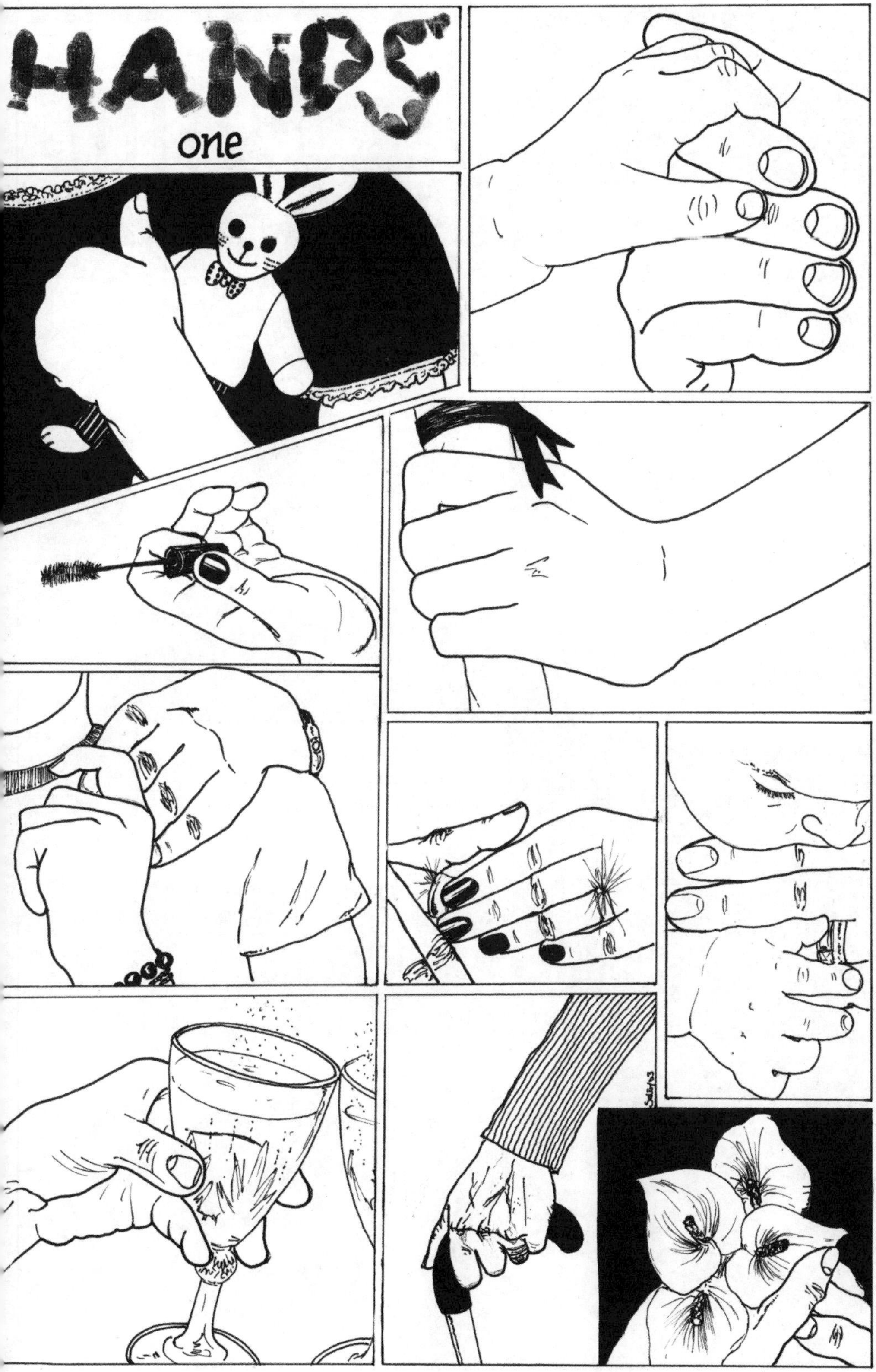
HANDS
one

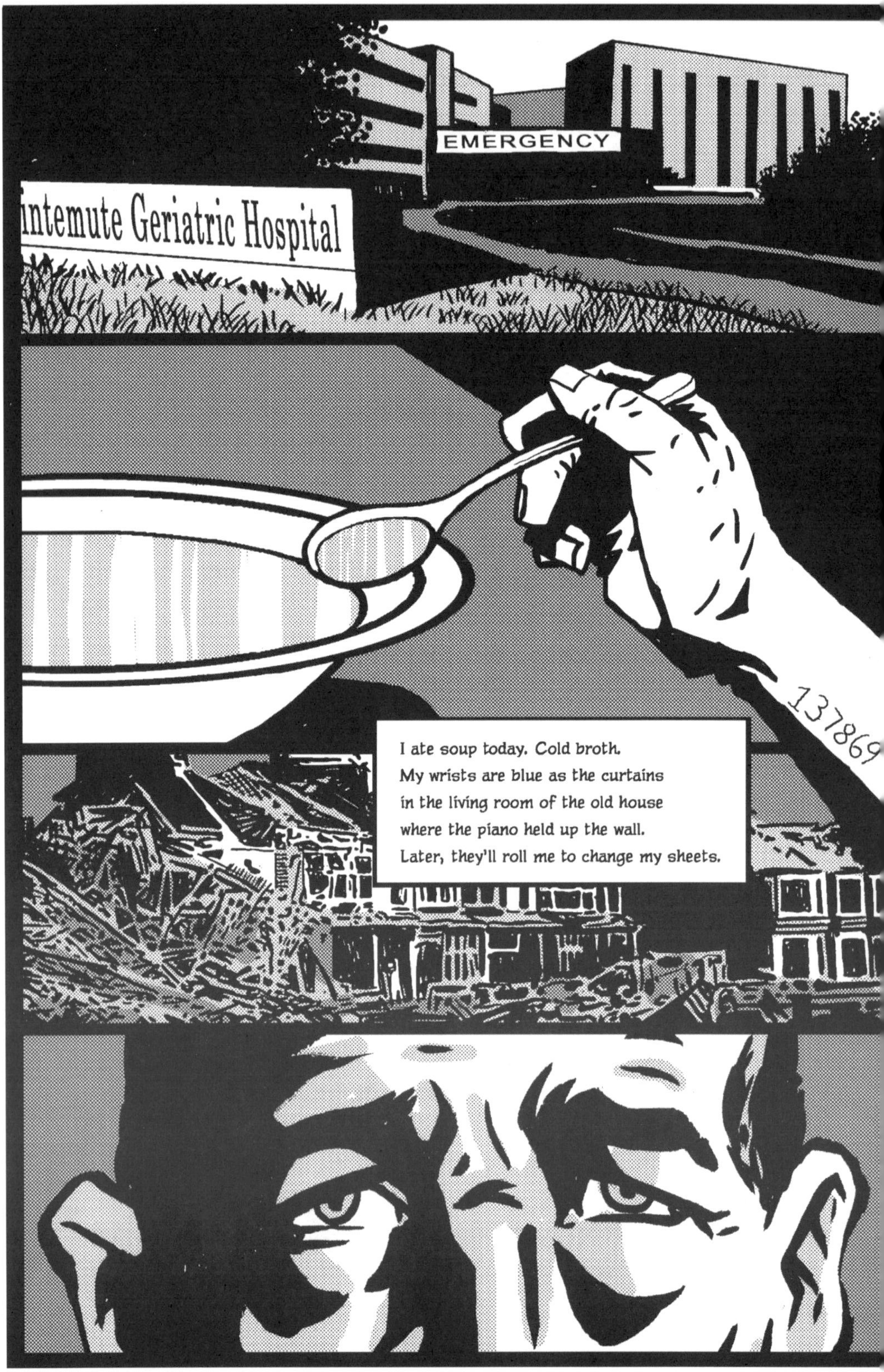
EMERGENCY
intemute Geriatric Hospital
137869
I ate soup today. Cold broth.
My wrists are blue as the curtains
in the living room of the old house
where the piano held up the wall.
Later, they'll roll me to change my sheets.

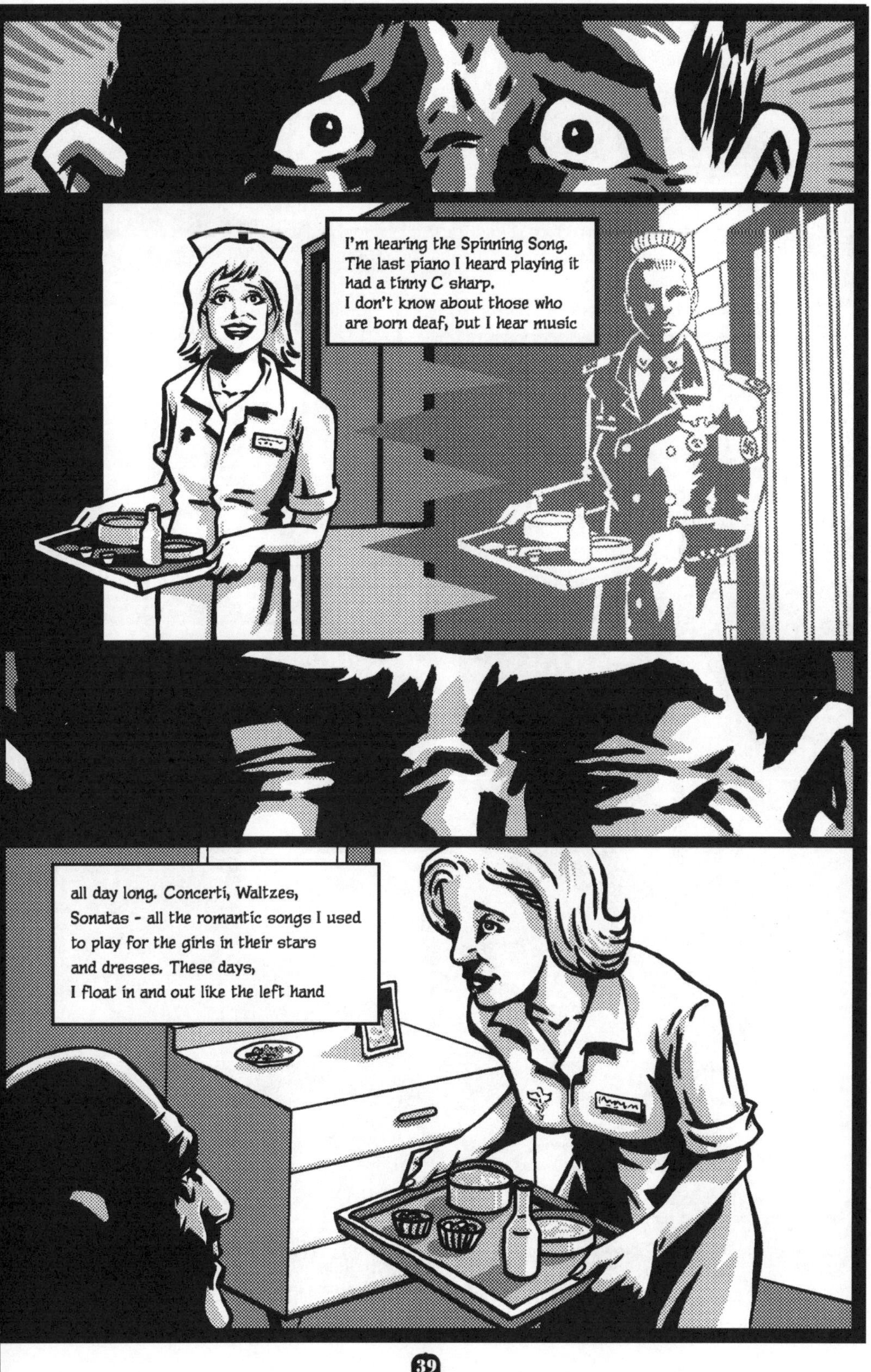
I'm hearing the Spinning Song. The last piano I heard playing it had a tinny C sharp. I don't know about those who are born deaf, but I hear music
all day long. Concerti, Waltzes, Sonatas - all the romantic songs I used to play for the girls in their stars and dresses. These days, I float in and out like the left hand

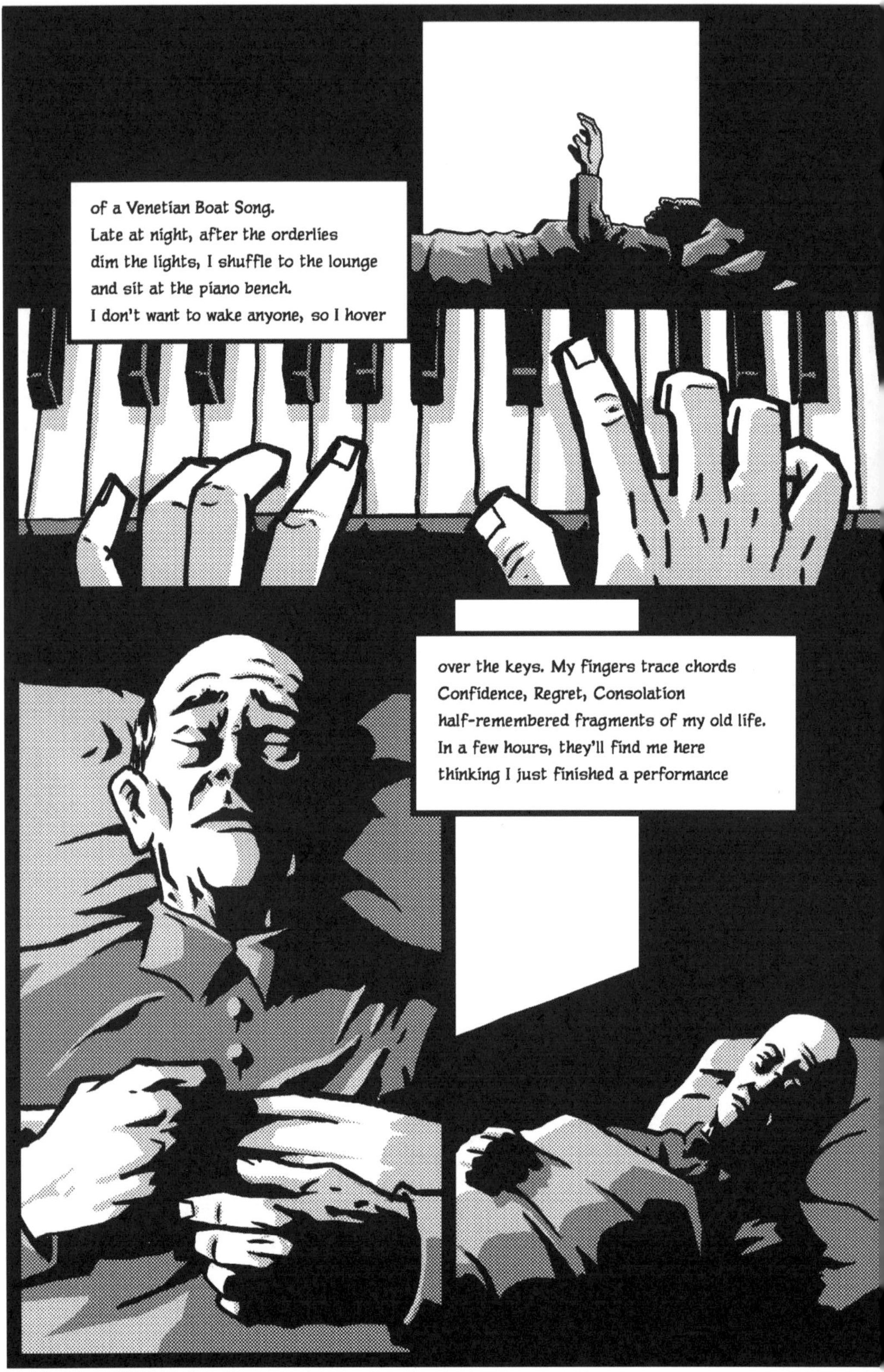
of a Venetian Boat Song.
Late at night, after the orderlies
dim the lights, I shuffle to the lounge
and sit at the piano bench.
I don't want to wake anyone, so I hover
over the keys. My fingers trace chords
Confidence, Regret, Consolation
half-remembered fragments of my old life.
In a few hours, they'll find me here
thinking I just finished a performance

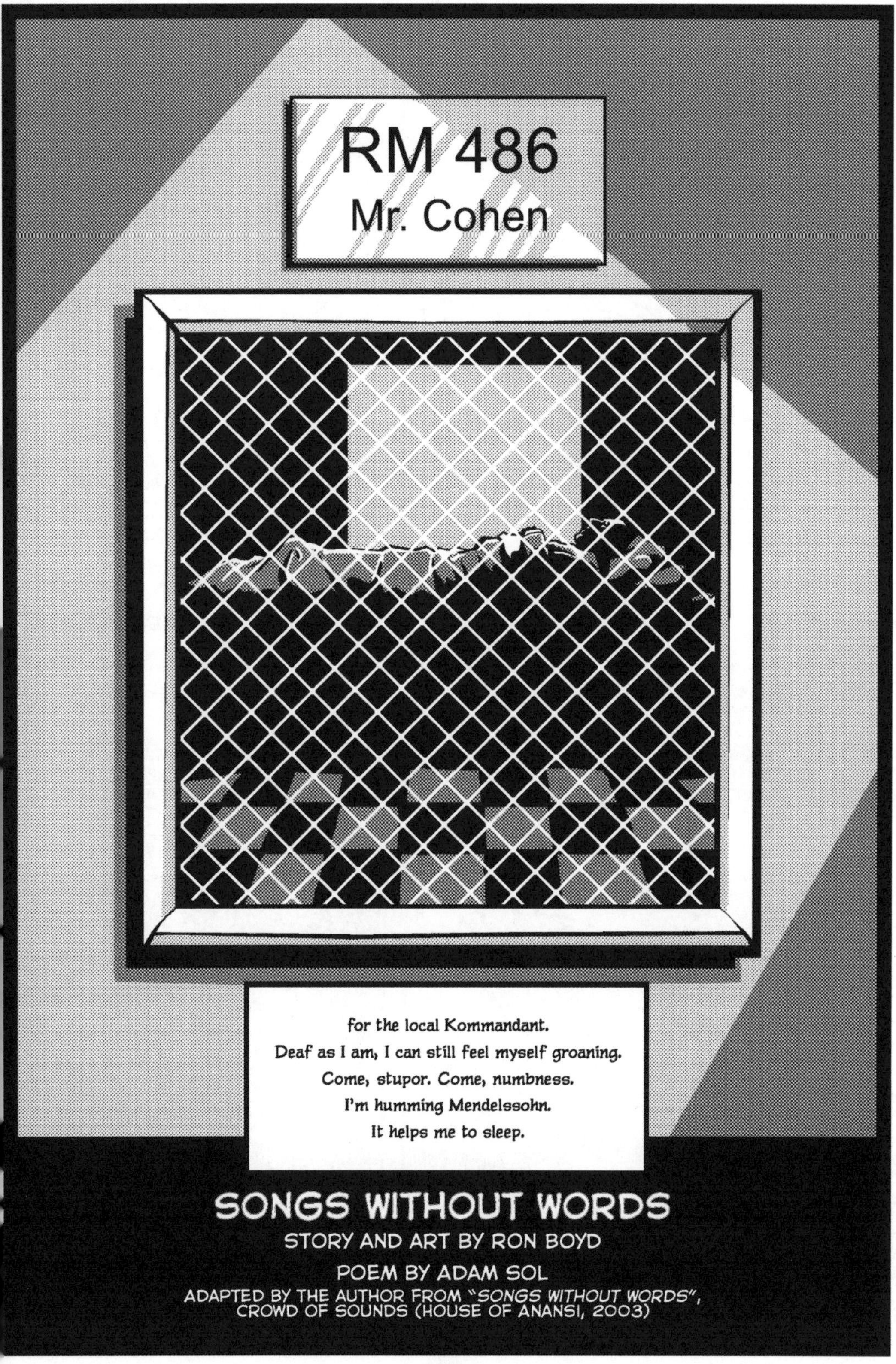

SONGS WITHOUT WORDS

STORY AND ART BY RON BOYD

POEM BY ADAM SOL

ADAPTED BY THE AUTHOR FROM "*SONGS WITHOUT WORDS*", CROWD OF SOUNDS (HOUSE OF ANANSI, 2003)

Le Cameleon Et Les Couleurs de la Vie

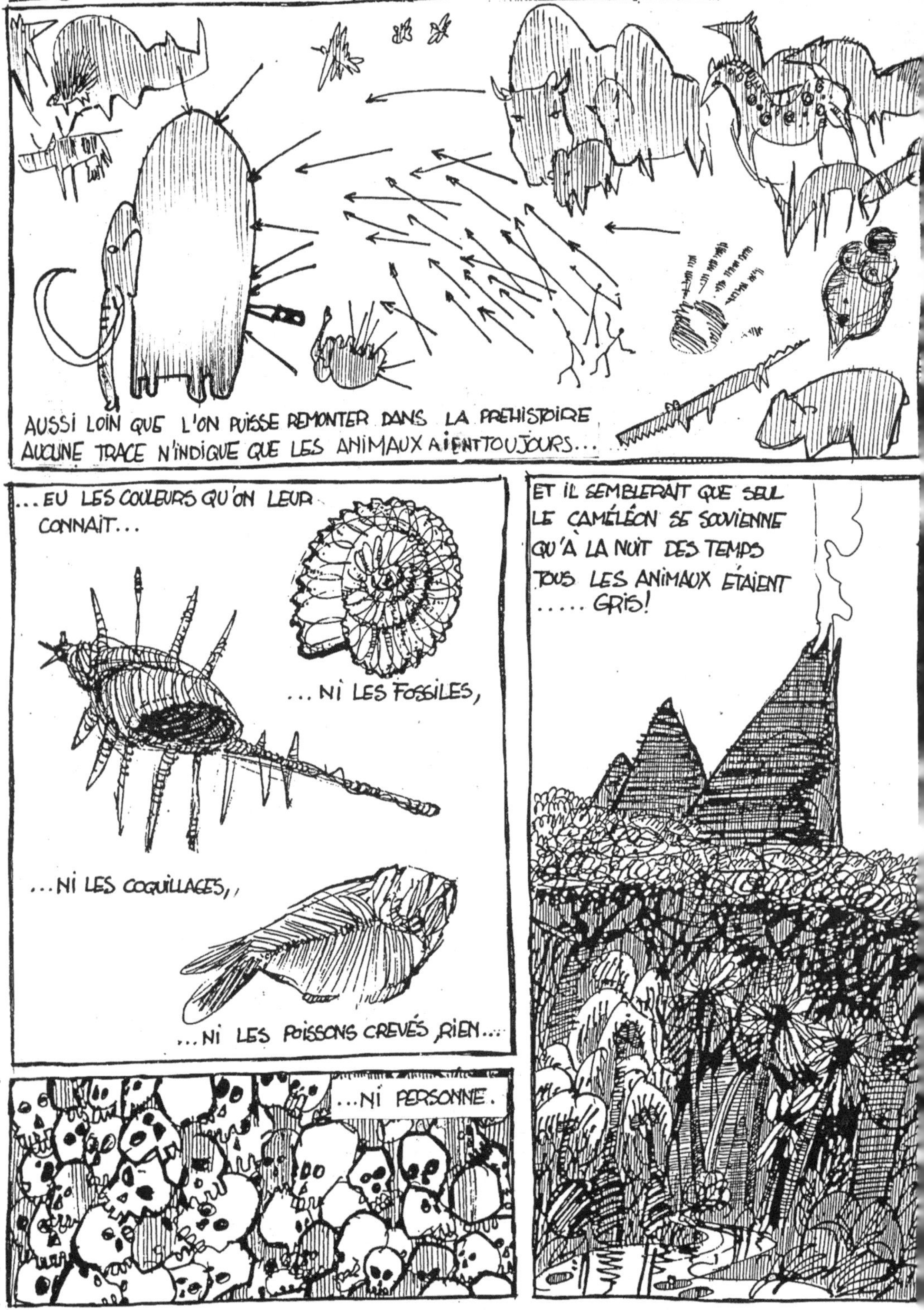

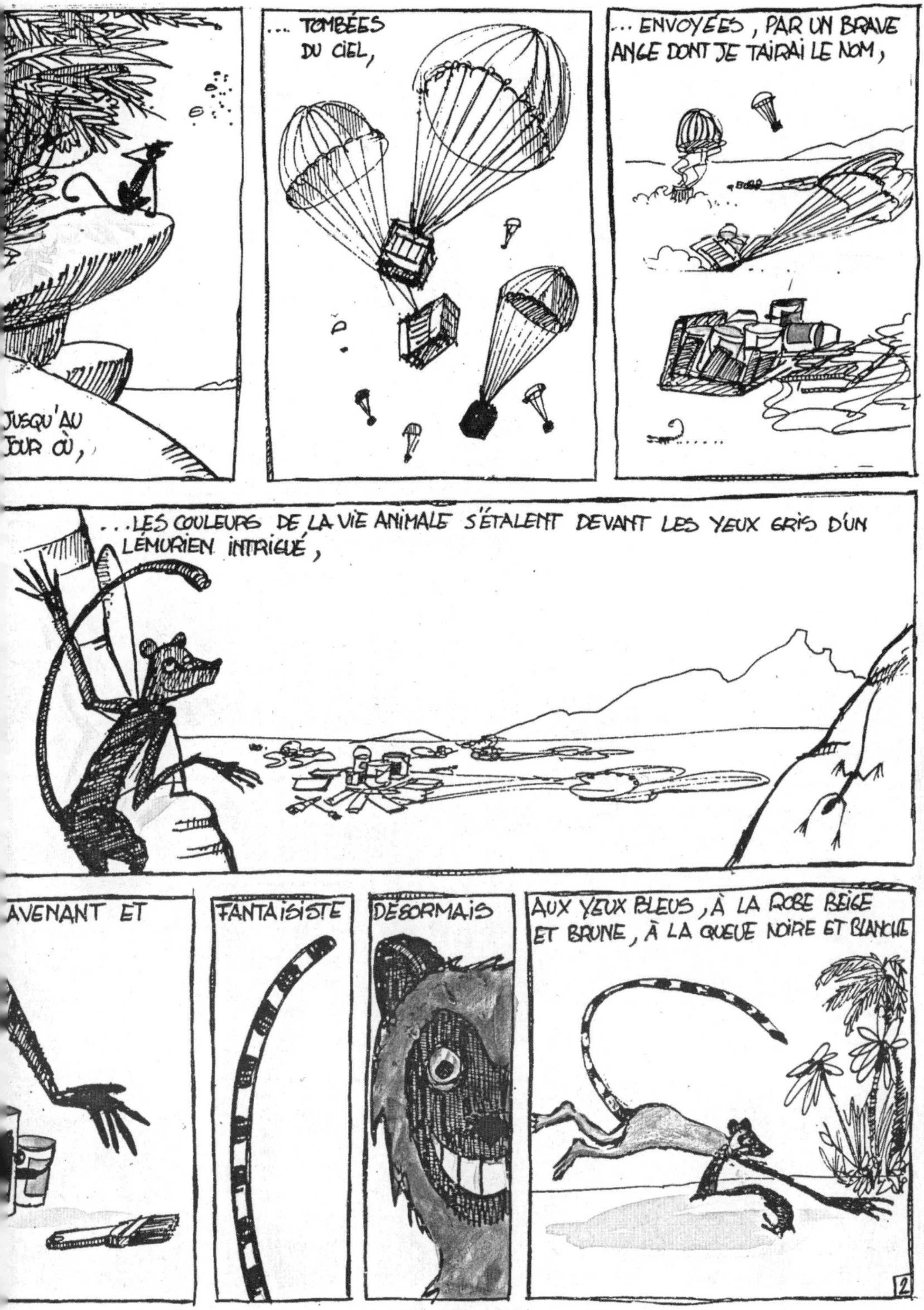
JUSQU'AU JOUR OÙ,
.... TOMBÉES DU CIEL,
... ENVOYÉES, PAR UN BRAVE ANGE DONT JE TAIRAI LE NOM,
...LES COULEURS DE LA VIE ANIMALE S'ÉTALENT DEVANT LES YEUX GRIS D'UN LÉMURIEN INTRIGUÉ,
AVENANT ET
FANTAISISTE
DÉSORMAIS
AUX YEUX BLEUS, À LA ROBE BEIGE ET BRUNE, À LA QUEUE NOIRE ET BLANCHE
2

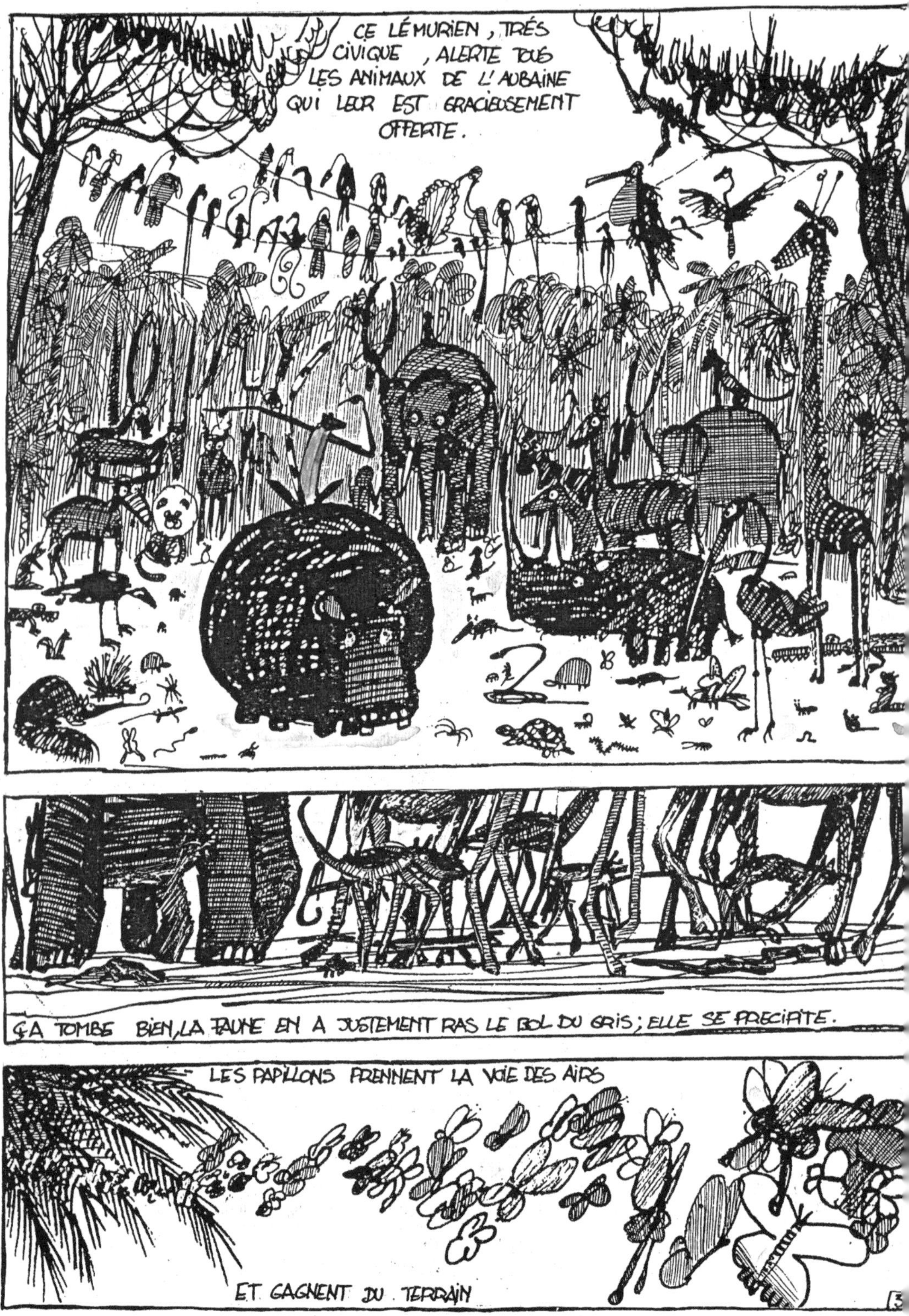
CE LÉMURIEN, TRÉS CIVIQUE, ALERTE TOUS LES ANIMAUX DE L'AUBAINE QUI LEUR EST GRACIEUSEMENT OFFERTE.
ÇA TOMBE BIEN, LA FAUNE EN A JUSTEMENT RAS LE BOL DU GRIS; ELLE SE PRECIPITE.
LES PAPILLONS PRENNENT LA VOIE DES AIRS
ET GAGNENT DU TERRAIN

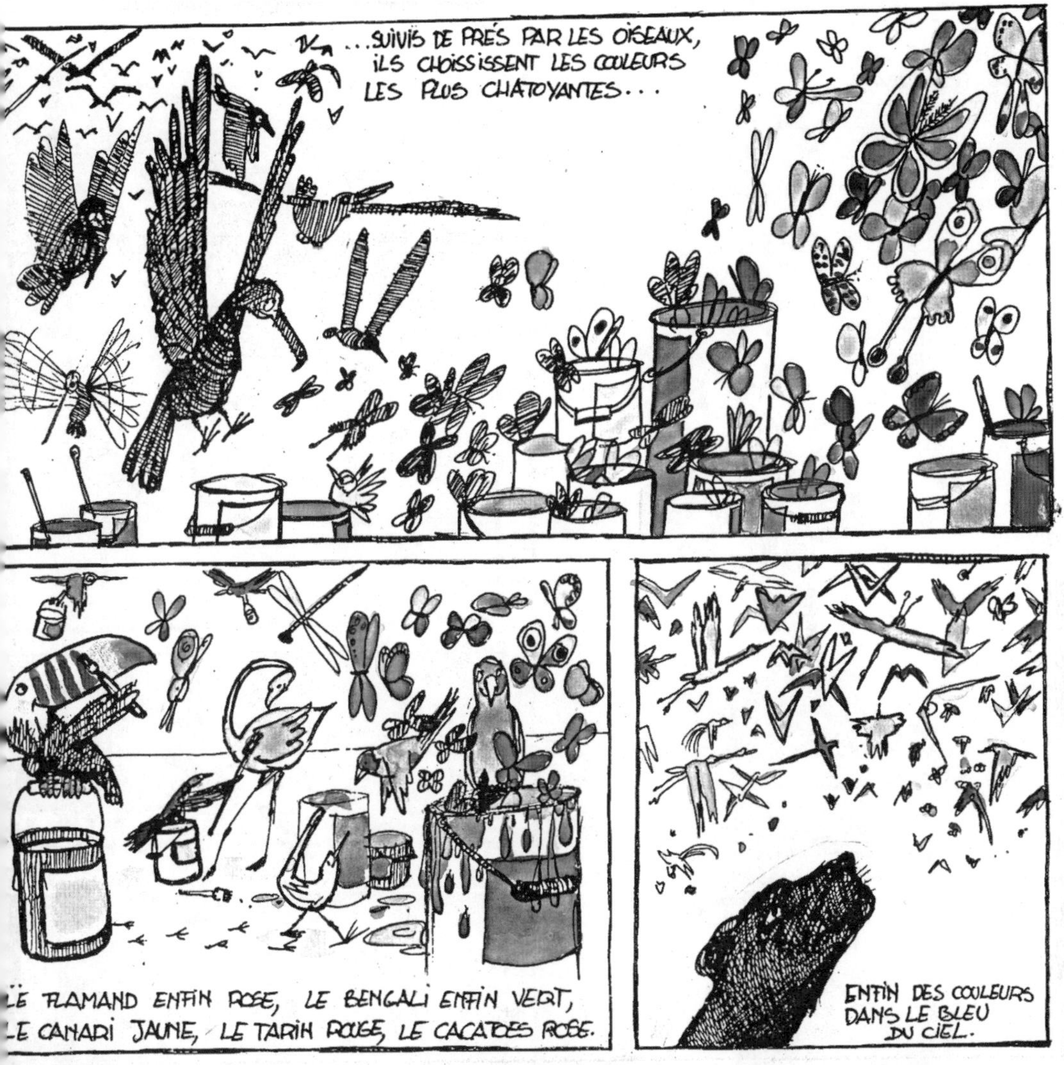
...SUIVIS DE PRÈS PAR LES OISEAUX,
ILS CHOISISSENT LES COULEURS
LES PLUS CHATOYANTES...
LE FLAMAND ENFIN ROSE, LE BENGALI ENFIN VERT,
LE CANARI JAUNE, LE TARIN ROUGE, LE CACATOES ROSE.
ENFIN DES COULEURS
DANS LE BLEU
DU CIEL.
AU SOL, ON HABILLE LE LEOPARD ET LE TIGRE PENDANT QUE LES GRENOUILLES SE
DÉBROUILLENT TOUTES SEULES SOUS LES YEUX DU MANDRILL.
4

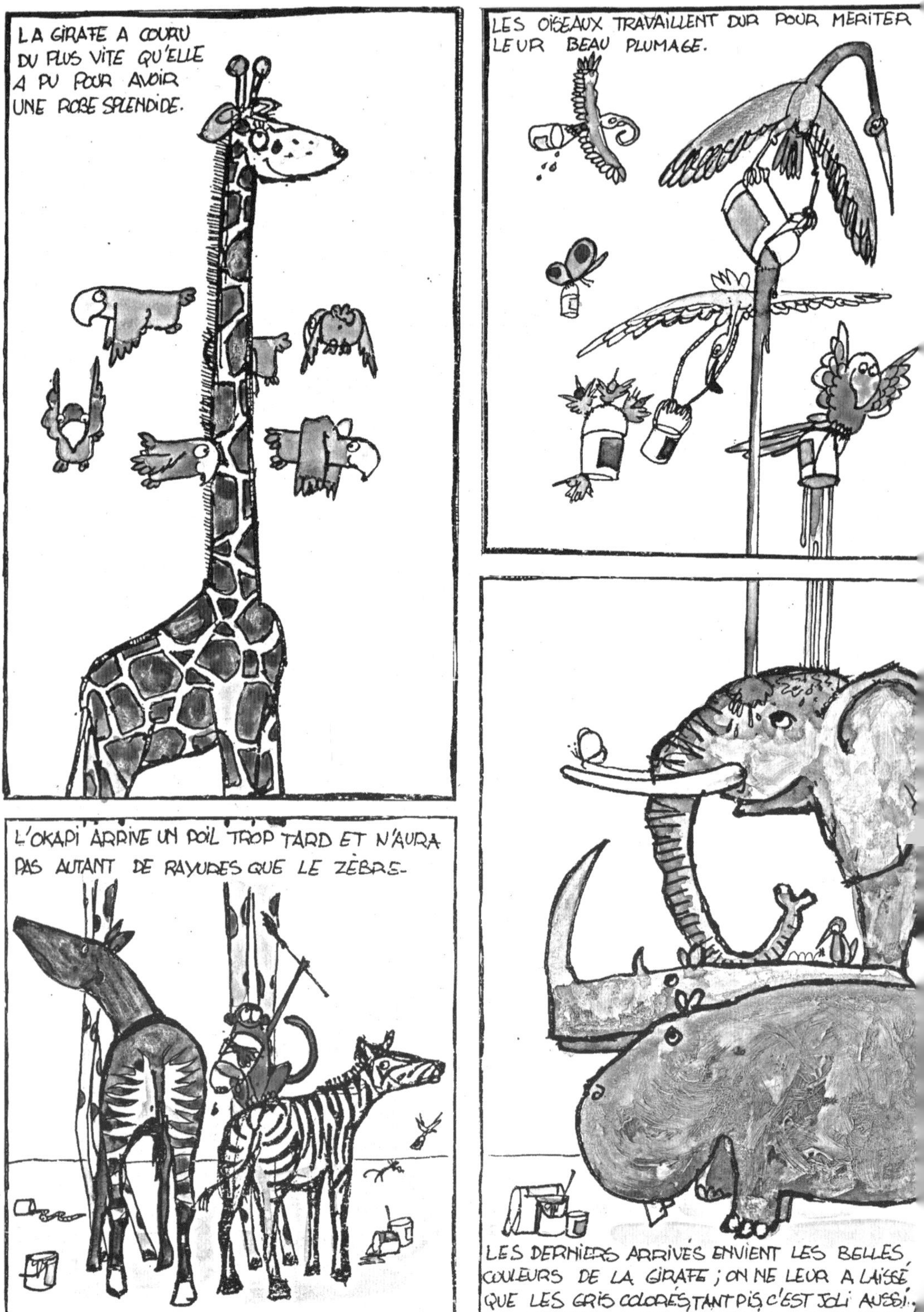
LA GIRAFE A COURU DU PLUS VITE QU'ELLE A PU POUR AVOIR UNE ROBE SPLENDIDE.
LES OISEAUX TRAVAILLENT DUR POUR MERITER LEUR BEAU PLUMAGE.
L'OKAPI ARRIVE UN POIL TROP TARD ET N'AURA PAS AUTANT DE RAYURES QUE LE ZÈBRE-
LES DERNIERS ARRIVÉS ENVIENT LES BELLES, COULEURS DE LA GIRAFE ; ON NE LEUR A LAISSÉ QUE LES GRIS COLORÉS, TANT PIS, C'EST JOLI AUSSI.

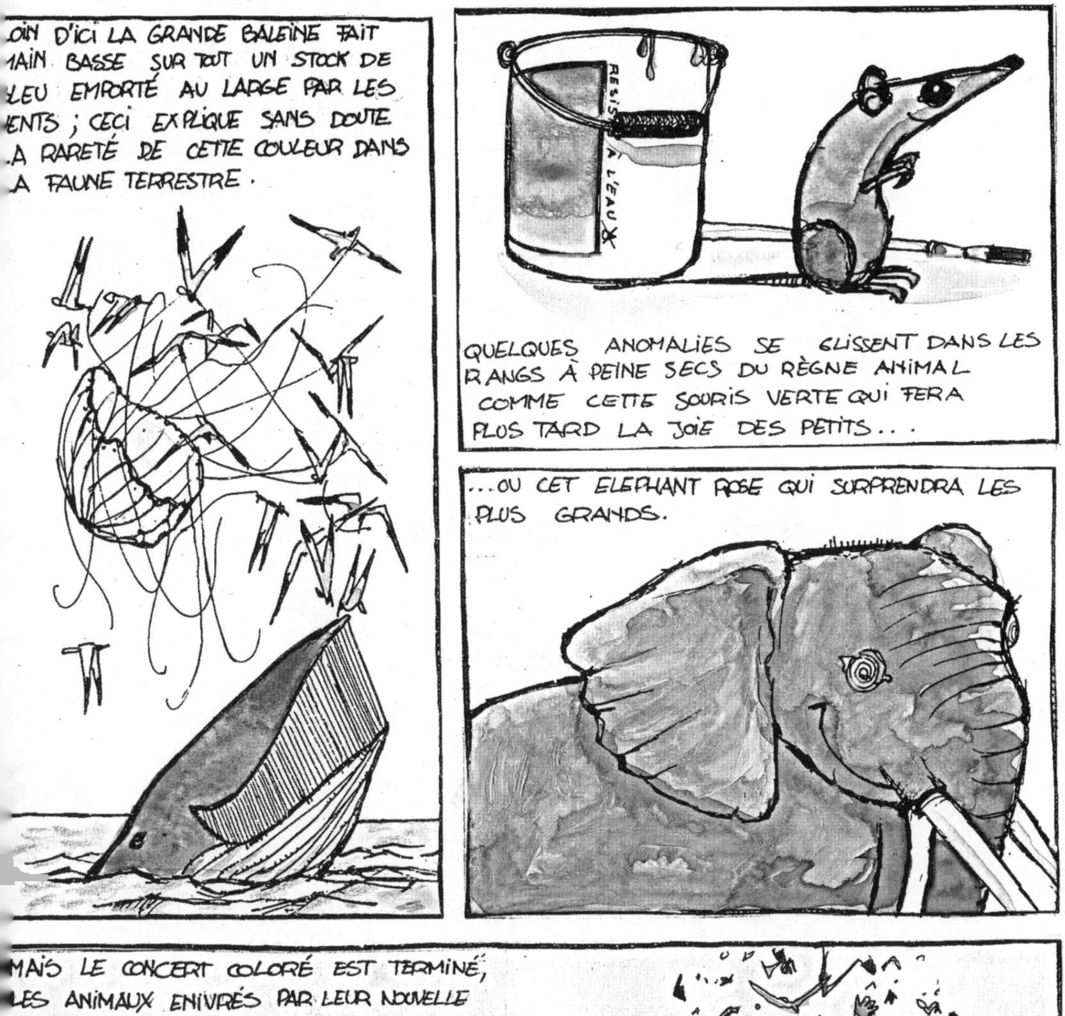
OIN D'ICI LA GRANDE BALEINE FAIT
AIN BASSE SUR TOUT UN STOCK DE
LEU EMPORTÉ AU LARGE PAR LES
ENTS ; CECI EXPLIQUE SANS DOUTE
A RARETÉ DE CETTE COULEUR DANS
A FAUNE TERRESTRE.
RESIS À L'EAU
QUELQUES ANOMALIES SE GLISSENT DANS LES RANGS À PEINE SECS DU RÈGNE ANIMAL COMME CETTE SOURIS VERTE QUI FERA PLUS TARD LA JOIE DES PETITS...
...OU CET ÉLÉPHANT ROSE QUI SURPRENDRA LES PLUS GRANDS.
MAIS LE CONCERT COLORÉ EST TERMINÉ, LES ANIMAUX ENIVRÉS PAR LEUR NOUVELLE ROBE, LEURS NOUVEAUX PELAGES, PLUMAGES OU ÉCAILLES SONT TOUS FOUS DE JOIE...
NON PAS TOUS; PERSONNE NE REMARQUE L'INDIVIDU QUI S'APPROCHE OUBLIÉ DE LA COURSE FOLLE AUX COULEURS, LE PLUS LENT D'ENTRE TOUS, LE DERNIER ENTRE LES DERNIERS, PLUS TRISTE ET PLUS GRIS QUE JAMAIS : LE CAMÉLÉON !
6

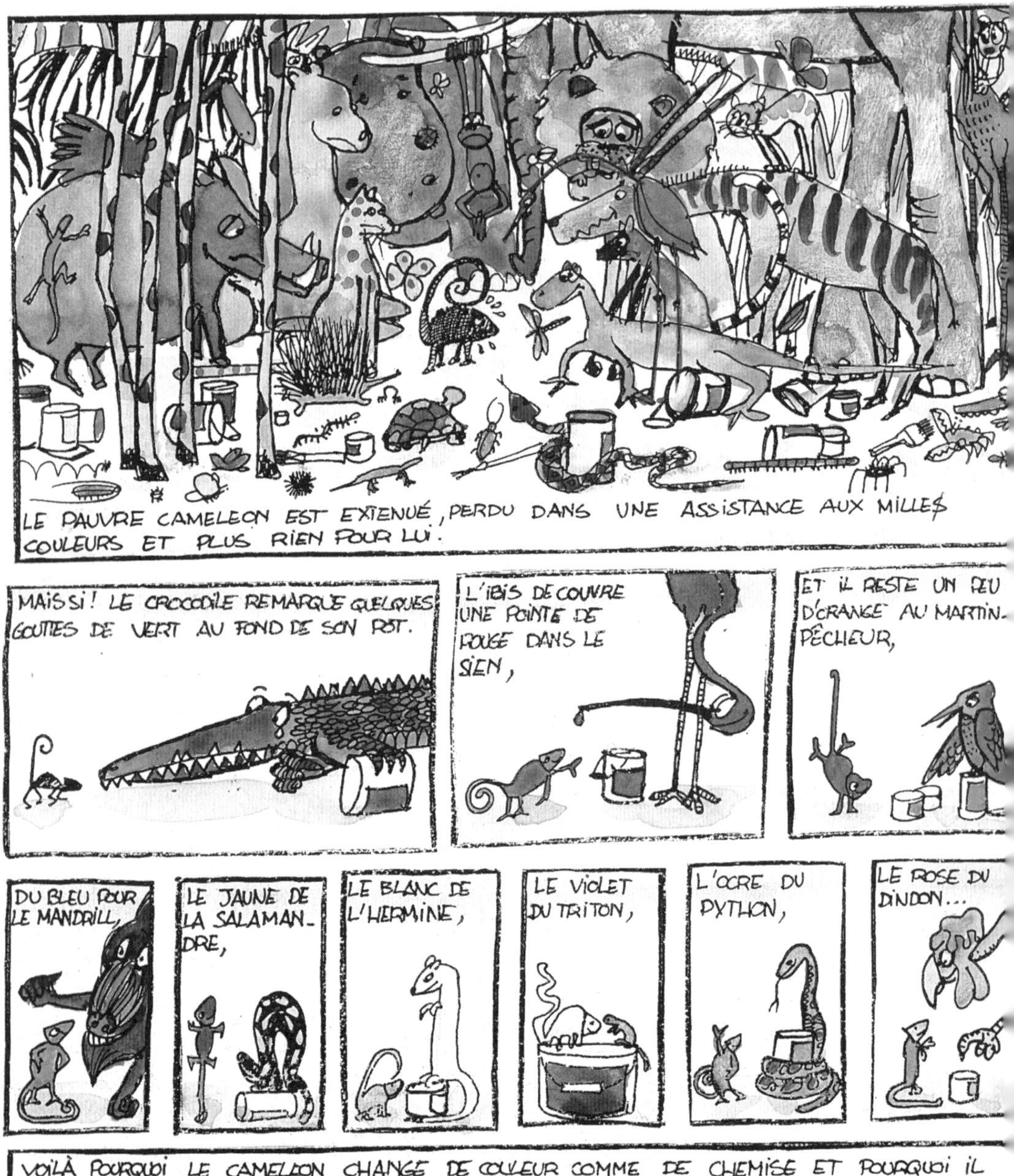
LE PAUVRE CAMELEON EST EXTENUÉ, PERDU DANS UNE ASSISTANCE AUX MILLES COULEURS ET PLUS RIEN POUR LUI.
MAIS SI ! LE CROCODILE REMARQUE QUELQUES GOUTTES DE VERT AU FOND DE SON POT.
L'IBIS DECOUVRE UNE POINTE DE ROUGE DANS LE SIEN,
ET IL RESTE UN PEU D'ORANGE AU MARTIN-PÊCHEUR,
DU BLEU POUR LE MANDRILL,
LE JAUNE DE LA SALAMANDRE,
LE BLANC DE L'HERMINE,
LE VIOLET DU TRITON,
L'OCRE DU PYTHON,
LE ROSE DU DINDON...
VOILÀ POURQUOI LE CAMELEON CHANGE DE COULEUR COMME DE CHEMISE ET POURQUOI IL EST LE SEUL À SE SOUVENIR QU'À LA NUIT DES TEMPS TOUS LES ANIMAUX ÉTAIENT GRIS.
FIN

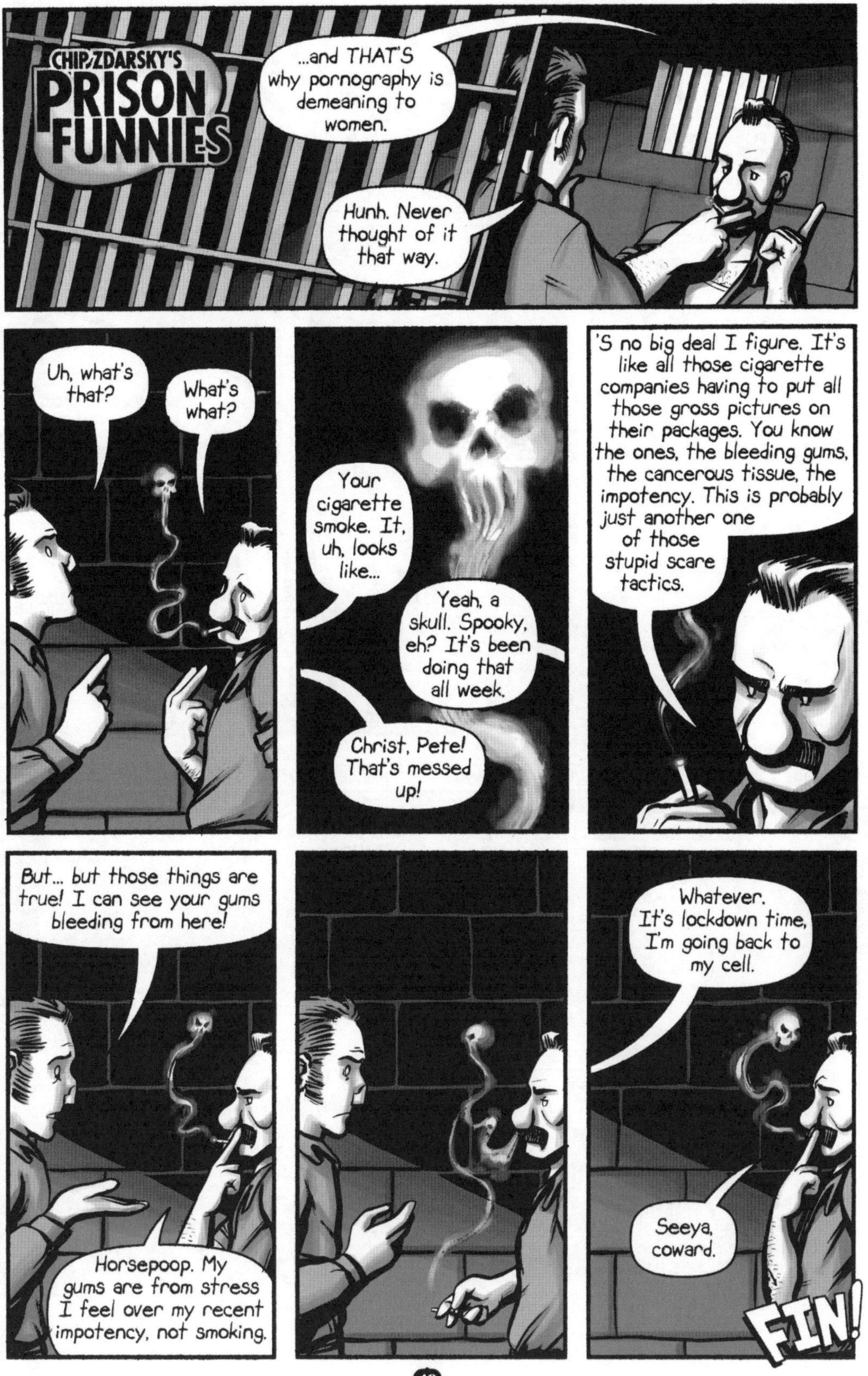
CHIP ZDARSKY'S
PRISON FUNNIES
...and THAT'S why pornography is demeaning to women.
Hunh. Never thought of it that way.
Uh, what's that?
What's what?
Your cigarette smoke. It, uh, looks like...
Yeah, a skull. Spooky, eh? It's been doing that all week.
Christ, Pete! That's messed up!
'S no big deal I figure. It's like all those cigarette companies having to put all those gross pictures on their packages. You know the ones, the bleeding gums, the cancerous tissue, the impotency. This is probably just another one of those stupid scare tactics.
But... but those things are true! I can see your gums bleeding from here!
Horsepoop. My gums are from stress I feel over my recent impotency, not smoking.
Whatever. It's lockdown time, I'm going back to my cell.
Seeya, coward.
FIN!

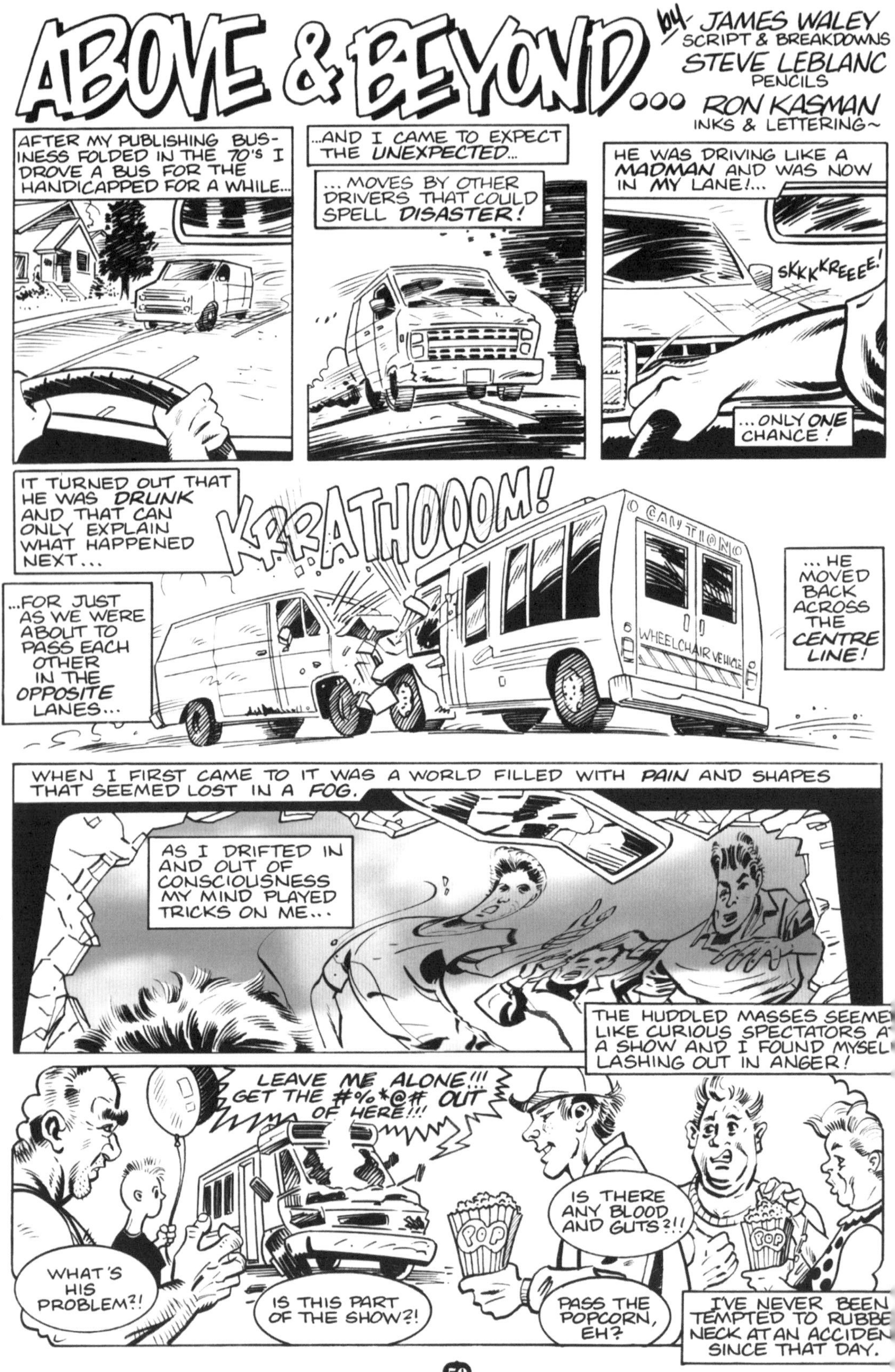
ABOVE & BEYOND...
by JAMES WALEY SCRIPT & BREAKDOWNS
STEVE LEBLANC PENCILS
RON KASMAN INKS & LETTERING~
AFTER MY PUBLISHING BUSINESS FOLDED IN THE 70'S I DROVE A BUS FOR THE HANDICAPPED FOR A WHILE...
...AND I CAME TO EXPECT THE UNEXPECTED...
...MOVES BY OTHER DRIVERS THAT COULD SPELL DISASTER!
HE WAS DRIVING LIKE A MADMAN AND WAS NOW IN MY LANE!...
SKKKKREEEE!
...ONLY ONE CHANCE!
IT TURNED OUT THAT HE WAS DRUNK AND THAT CAN ONLY EXPLAIN WHAT HAPPENED NEXT...
KRRATHOOOM!
...FOR JUST AS WE WERE ABOUT TO PASS EACH OTHER IN THE OPPOSITE LANES...
...HE MOVED BACK ACROSS THE CENTRE LINE!
CAUTION
WHEELCHAIR VEHICLE
WHEN I FIRST CAME TO IT WAS A WORLD FILLED WITH PAIN AND SHAPES THAT SEEMED LOST IN A FOG.
AS I DRIFTED IN AND OUT OF CONSCIOUSNESS MY MIND PLAYED TRICKS ON ME...
THE HUDDLED MASSES SEEME LIKE CURIOUS SPECTATORS A A SHOW AND I FOUND MYSEL LASHING OUT IN ANGER!
LEAVE ME ALONE!!! GET THE #%*@# OUT OF HERE!!!
WHAT'S HIS PROBLEM?!
IS THIS PART OF THE SHOW?!
IS THERE ANY BLOOD AND GUTS?!!
PASS THE POPCORN, EH?
POP
I'VE NEVER BEEN TEMPTED TO RUBBE NECK AT AN ACCIDEN SINCE THAT DAY.

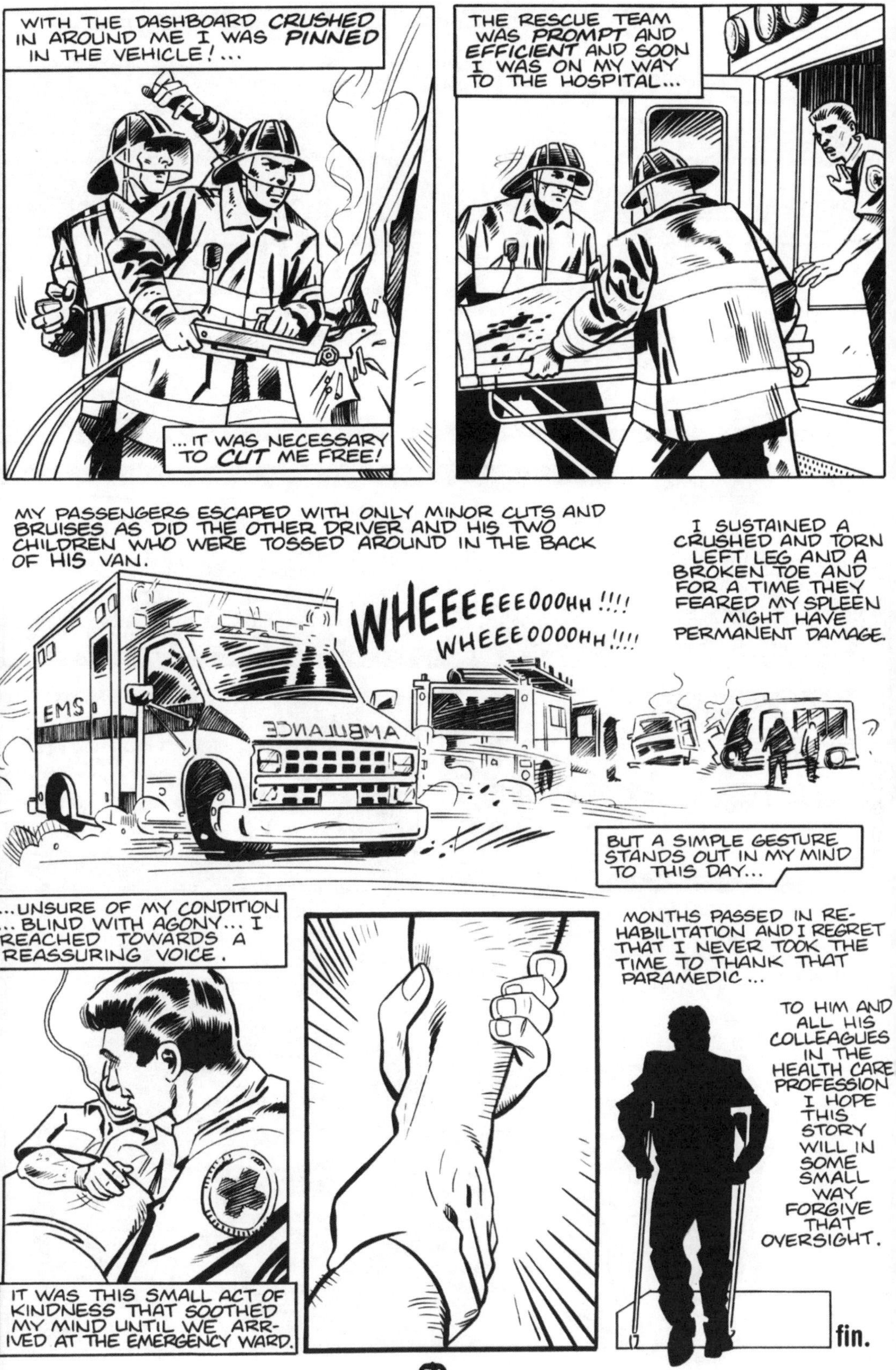
WITH THE DASHBOARD CRUSHED IN AROUND ME I WAS PINNED IN THE VEHICLE!...
...IT WAS NECESSARY TO CUT ME FREE!
THE RESCUE TEAM WAS PROMPT AND EFFICIENT AND SOON I WAS ON MY WAY TO THE HOSPITAL...
MY PASSENGERS ESCAPED WITH ONLY MINOR CUTS AND BRUISES AS DID THE OTHER DRIVER AND HIS TWO CHILDREN WHO WERE TOSSED AROUND IN THE BACK OF HIS VAN.
I SUSTAINED A CRUSHED AND TORN LEFT LEG AND A BROKEN TOE AND FOR A TIME THEY FEARED MY SPLEEN MIGHT HAVE PERMANENT DAMAGE.
WHEEEEEEEOOOHH!!!!
WHEEEOOOOHH!!!!
EMS
AMBULANCE
BUT A SIMPLE GESTURE STANDS OUT IN MY MIND TO THIS DAY...
...UNSURE OF MY CONDITION ...BLIND WITH AGONY... I REACHED TOWARDS A REASSURING VOICE.
IT WAS THIS SMALL ACT OF KINDNESS THAT SOOTHED MY MIND UNTIL WE ARRIVED AT THE EMERGENCY WARD.
MONTHS PASSED IN REHABILITATION AND I REGRET THAT I NEVER TOOK THE TIME TO THANK THAT PARAMEDIC...
TO HIM AND ALL HIS COLLEAGUES IN THE HEALTH CARE PROFESSION I HOPE THIS STORY WILL IN SOME SMALL WAY FORGIVE THAT OVERSIGHT.
fin.

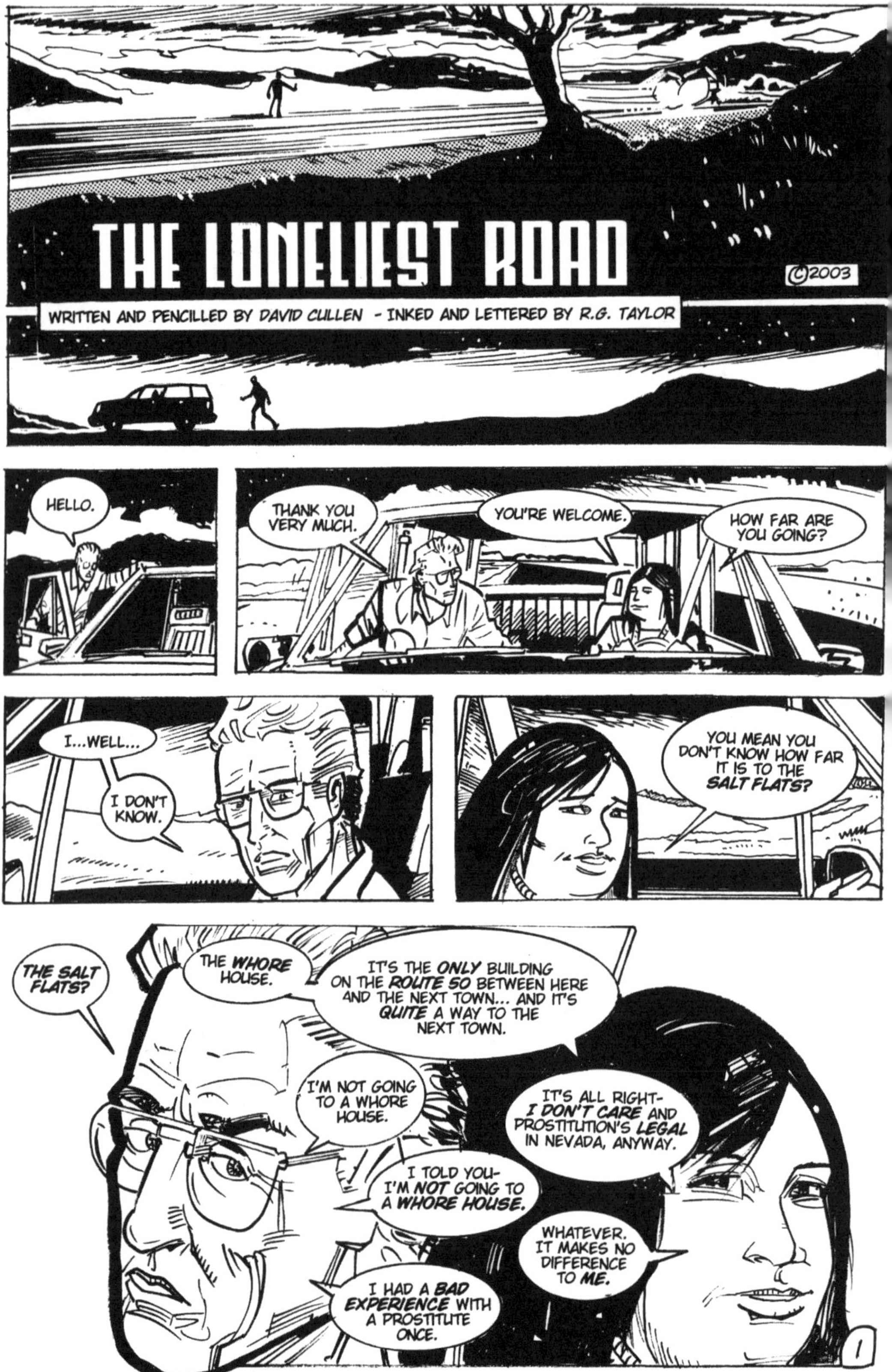
THE LONELIEST ROAD
©2003
WRITTEN AND PENCILLED BY DAVID CULLEN - INKED AND LETTERED BY R.G. TAYLOR
HELLO.
THANK YOU VERY MUCH.
YOU'RE WELCOME.
HOW FAR ARE YOU GOING?
I...WELL...
I DON'T KNOW.
YOU MEAN YOU DON'T KNOW HOW FAR IT IS TO THE SALT FLATS?
THE SALT FLATS?
THE WHORE HOUSE.
IT'S THE ONLY BUILDING ON THE ROUTE 50 BETWEEN HERE AND THE NEXT TOWN... AND IT'S QUITE A WAY TO THE NEXT TOWN.
I'M NOT GOING TO A WHORE HOUSE.
IT'S ALL RIGHT- I DON'T CARE AND PROSTITUTION'S LEGAL IN NEVADA, ANYWAY.
I TOLD YOU- I'M NOT GOING TO A WHORE HOUSE.
WHATEVER. IT MAKES NO DIFFERENCE TO ME.
I HAD A BAD EXPERIENCE WITH A PROSTITUTE ONCE.
1

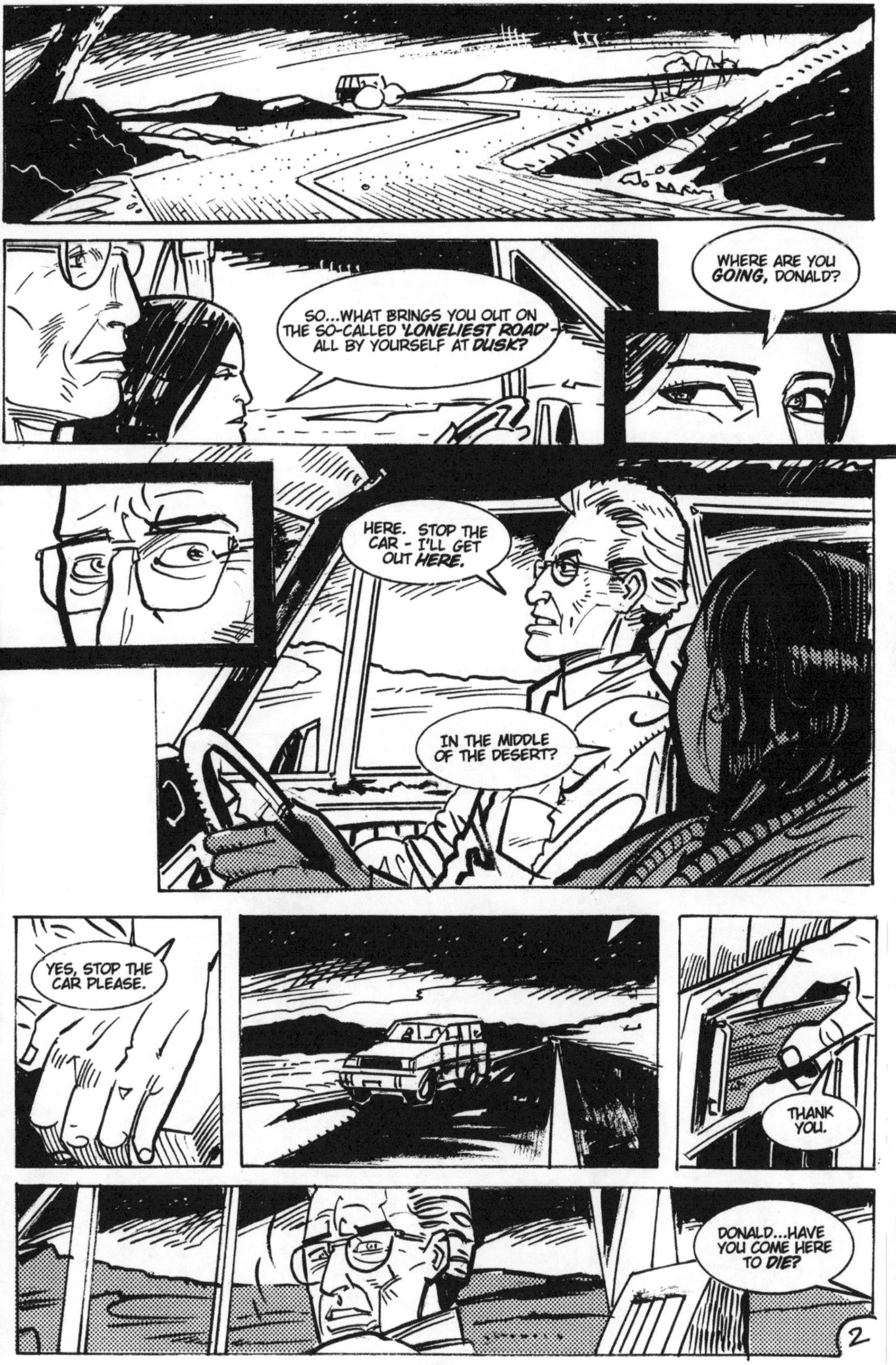

SO...WHAT BRINGS YOU OUT ON THE SO-CALLED 'LONELIEST ROAD' ALL BY YOURSELF AT DUSK?
WHERE ARE YOU GOING, DONALD?
HERE. STOP THE CAR - I'LL GET OUT HERE.
IN THE MIDDLE OF THE DESERT?
YES, STOP THE CAR PLEASE.
THANK YOU.
DONALD...HAVE YOU COME HERE TO DIE?
2

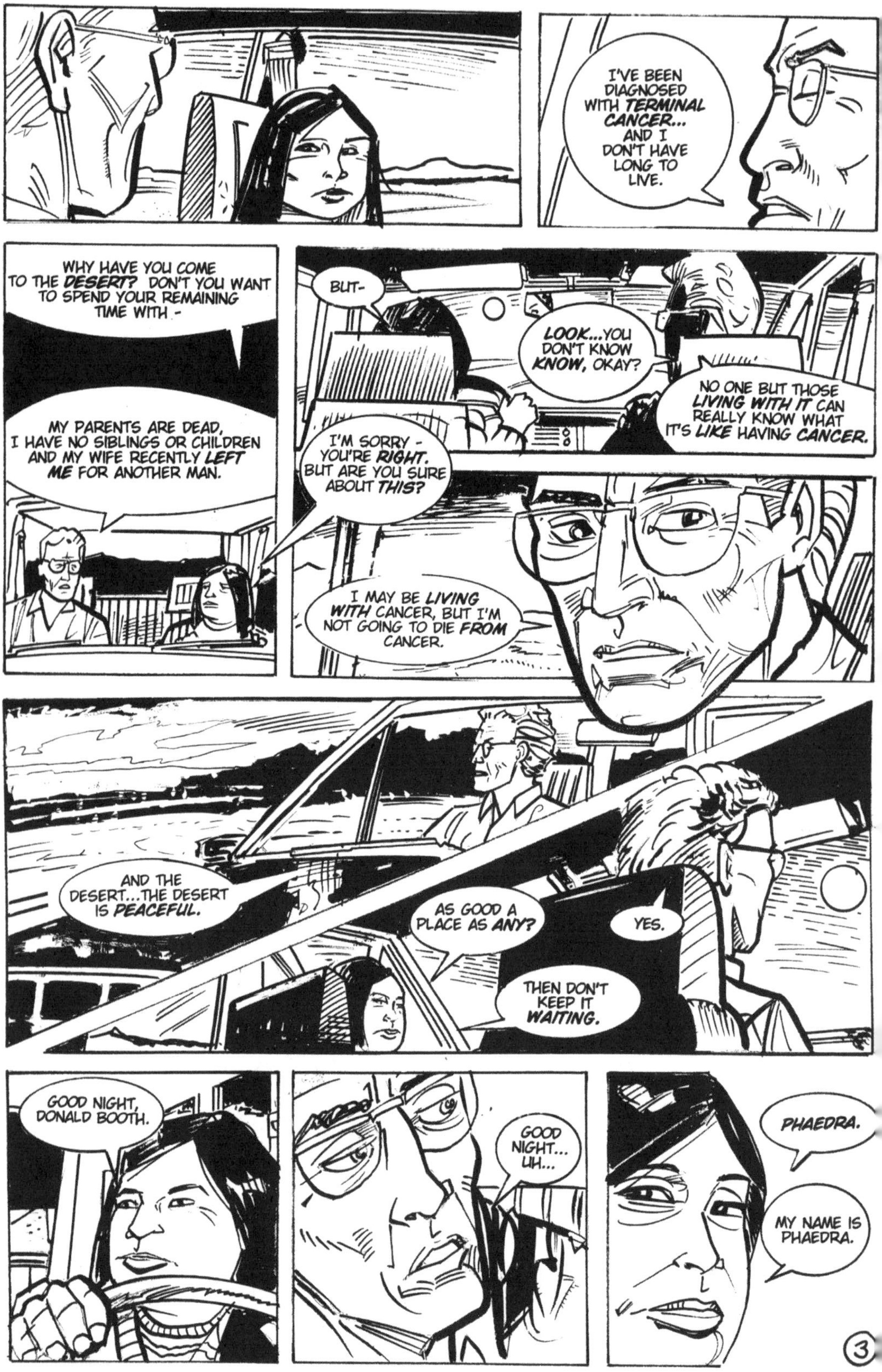
I'VE BEEN DIAGNOSED WITH TERMINAL CANCER... AND I DON'T HAVE LONG TO LIVE.
WHY HAVE YOU COME TO THE DESERT? DON'T YOU WANT TO SPEND YOUR REMAINING TIME WITH -
MY PARENTS ARE DEAD, I HAVE NO SIBLINGS OR CHILDREN AND MY WIFE RECENTLY LEFT ME FOR ANOTHER MAN.
BUT-
LOOK...YOU DON'T KNOW KNOW, OKAY?
NO ONE BUT THOSE LIVING WITH IT CAN REALLY KNOW WHAT IT'S LIKE HAVING CANCER.
I'M SORRY - YOU'RE RIGHT. BUT ARE YOU SURE ABOUT THIS?
I MAY BE LIVING WITH CANCER, BUT I'M NOT GOING TO DIE FROM CANCER.
AND THE DESERT...THE DESERT IS PEACEFUL.
AS GOOD A PLACE AS ANY?
YES.
THEN DON'T KEEP IT WAITING.
GOOD NIGHT, DONALD BOOTH.
GOOD NIGHT... UH...
PHAEDRA.
MY NAME IS PHAEDRA.
3

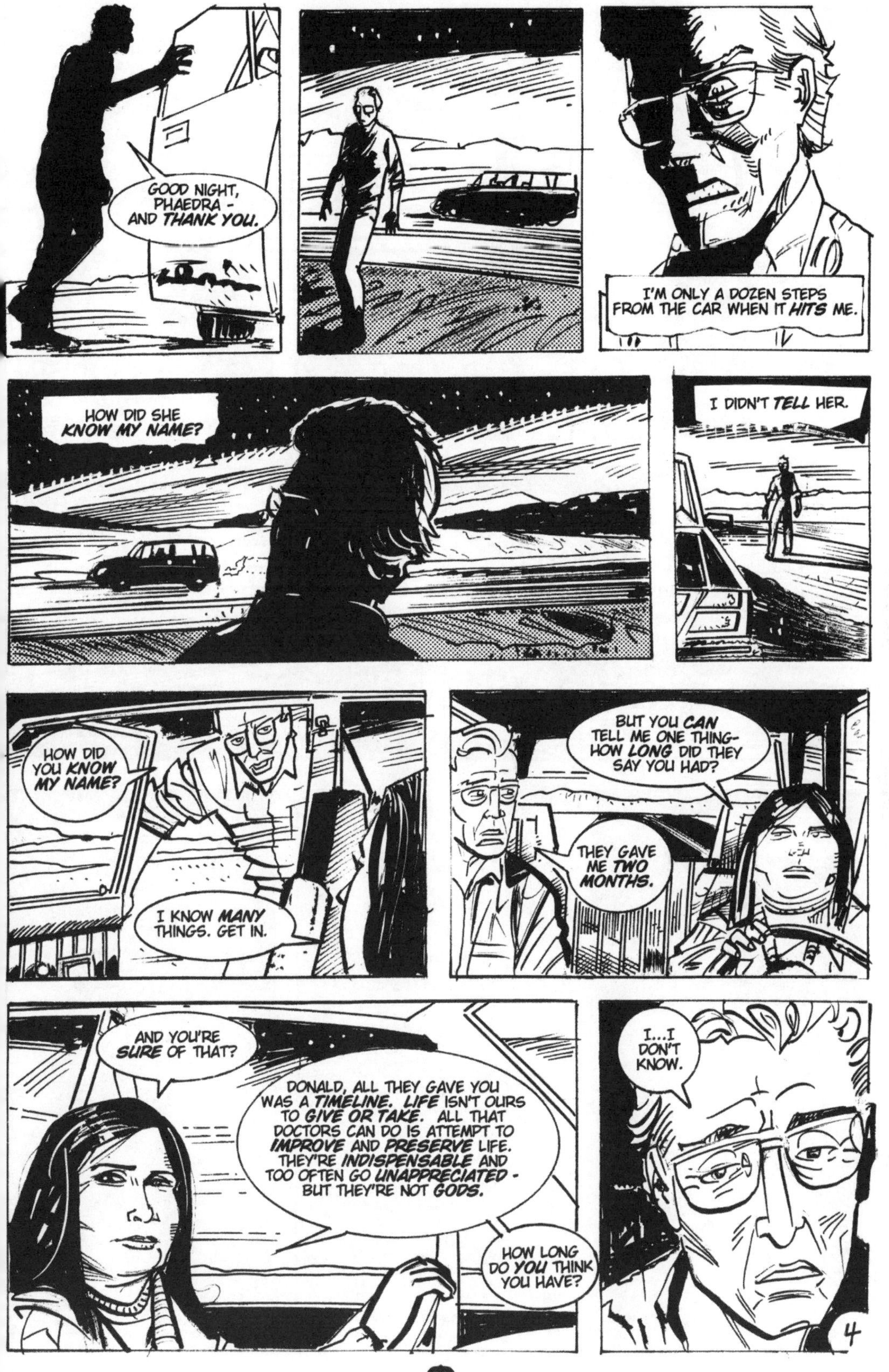
GOOD NIGHT, PHAEDRA - AND THANK YOU.
I'M ONLY A DOZEN STEPS FROM THE CAR WHEN IT HITS ME.
HOW DID SHE KNOW MY NAME?
I DIDN'T TELL HER.
HOW DID YOU KNOW MY NAME?
I KNOW MANY THINGS. GET IN.
BUT YOU CAN TELL ME ONE THING- HOW LONG DID THEY SAY YOU HAD?
THEY GAVE ME TWO MONTHS.
AND YOU'RE SURE OF THAT?
DONALD, ALL THEY GAVE YOU WAS A TIMELINE. LIFE ISN'T OURS TO GIVE OR TAKE. ALL THAT DOCTORS CAN DO IS ATTEMPT TO IMPROVE AND PRESERVE LIFE. THEY'RE INDISPENSABLE AND TOO OFTEN GO UNAPPRECIATED - BUT THEY'RE NOT GODS.
HOW LONG DO YOU THINK YOU HAVE?
I...I DON'T KNOW.
4

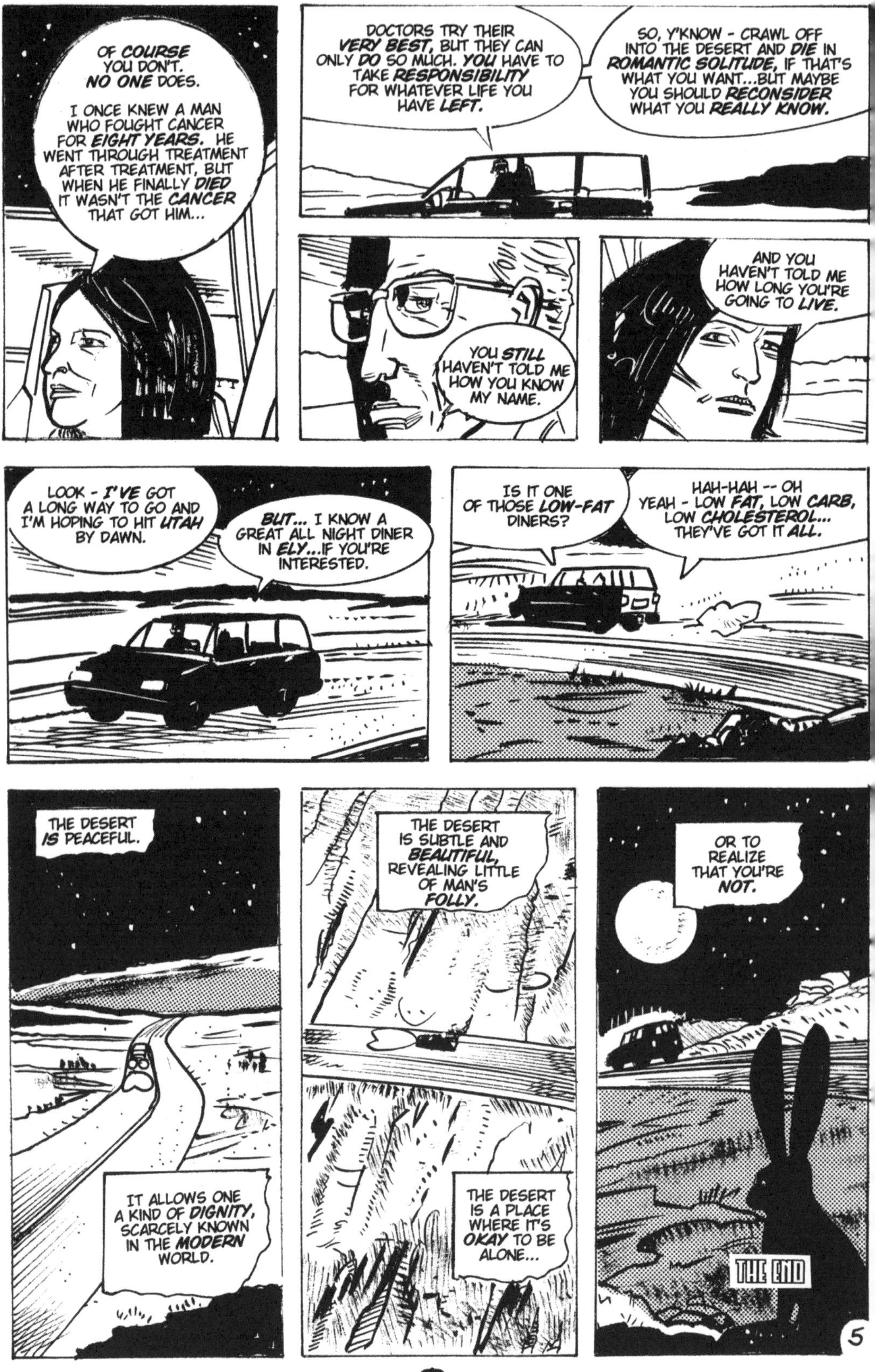

OF COURSE YOU DON'T. NO ONE DOES.
I ONCE KNEW A MAN WHO FOUGHT CANCER FOR EIGHT YEARS. HE WENT THROUGH TREATMENT AFTER TREATMENT, BUT WHEN HE FINALLY DIED IT WASN'T THE CANCER THAT GOT HIM...
DOCTORS TRY THEIR VERY BEST, BUT THEY CAN ONLY DO SO MUCH. YOU HAVE TO TAKE RESPONSIBILITY FOR WHATEVER LIFE YOU HAVE LEFT.
SO, Y'KNOW - CRAWL OFF INTO THE DESERT AND DIE IN ROMANTIC SOLITUDE, IF THAT'S WHAT YOU WANT...BUT MAYBE YOU SHOULD RECONSIDER WHAT YOU REALLY KNOW.
YOU STILL HAVEN'T TOLD ME HOW YOU KNOW MY NAME.
AND YOU HAVEN'T TOLD ME HOW LONG YOU'RE GOING TO LIVE.
LOOK - I'VE GOT A LONG WAY TO GO AND I'M HOPING TO HIT UTAH BY DAWN.
BUT... I KNOW A GREAT ALL NIGHT DINER IN ELY...IF YOU'RE INTERESTED.
IS IT ONE OF THOSE LOW-FAT DINERS?
HAH-HAH -- OH YEAH - LOW FAT, LOW CARB, LOW CHOLESTEROL... THEY'VE GOT IT ALL.
THE DESERT IS PEACEFUL.
IT ALLOWS ONE A KIND OF DIGNITY, SCARCELY KNOWN IN THE MODERN WORLD.
THE DESERT IS SUBTLE AND BEAUTIFUL, REVEALING LITTLE OF MAN'S FOLLY.
THE DESERT IS A PLACE WHERE IT'S OKAY TO BE ALONE...
OR TO REALIZE THAT YOU'RE NOT.
THE END
5

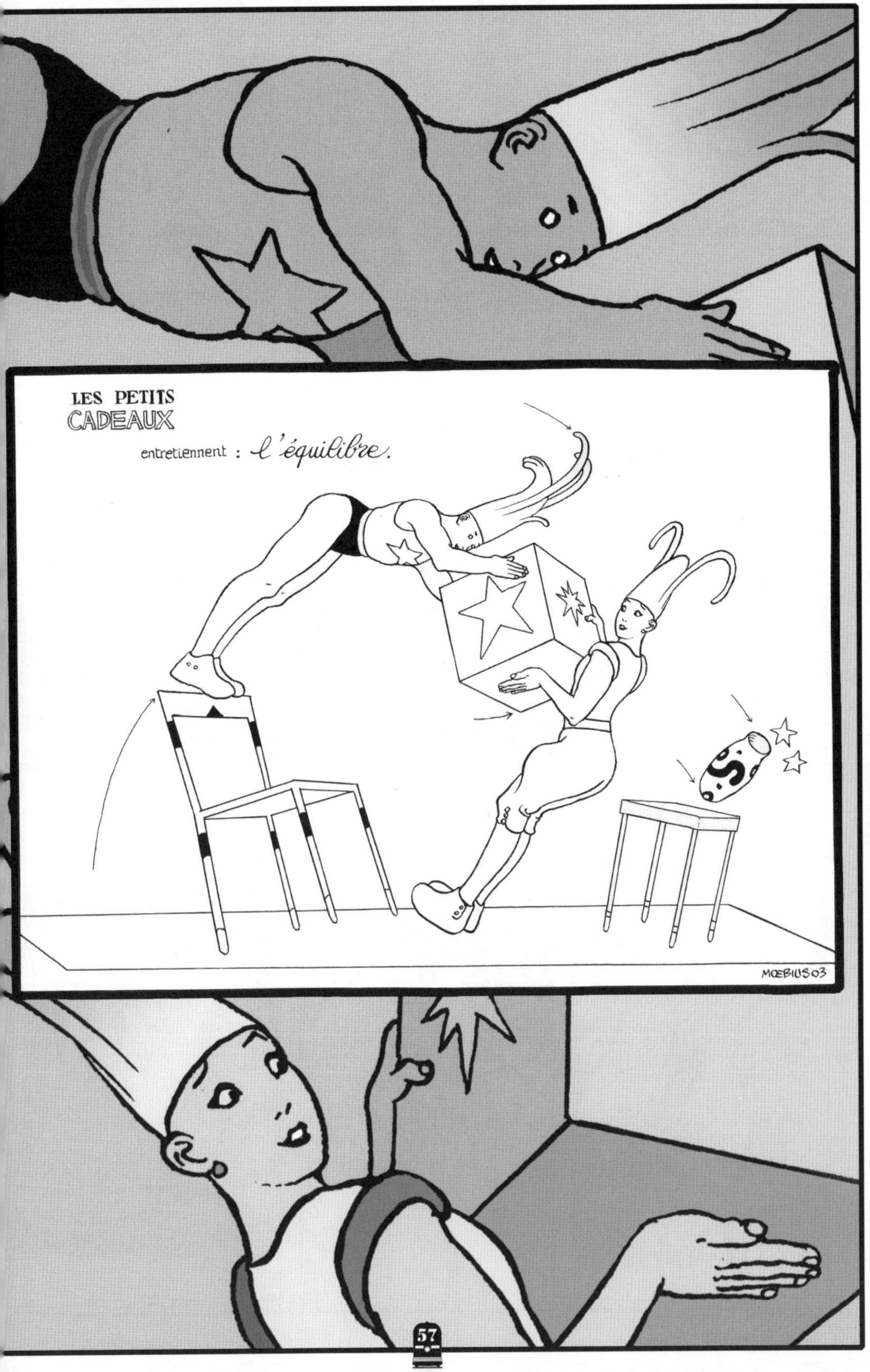

LES PETITS
CADEAUX
entretiennent : l'équilibre.
MŒBIUS 03

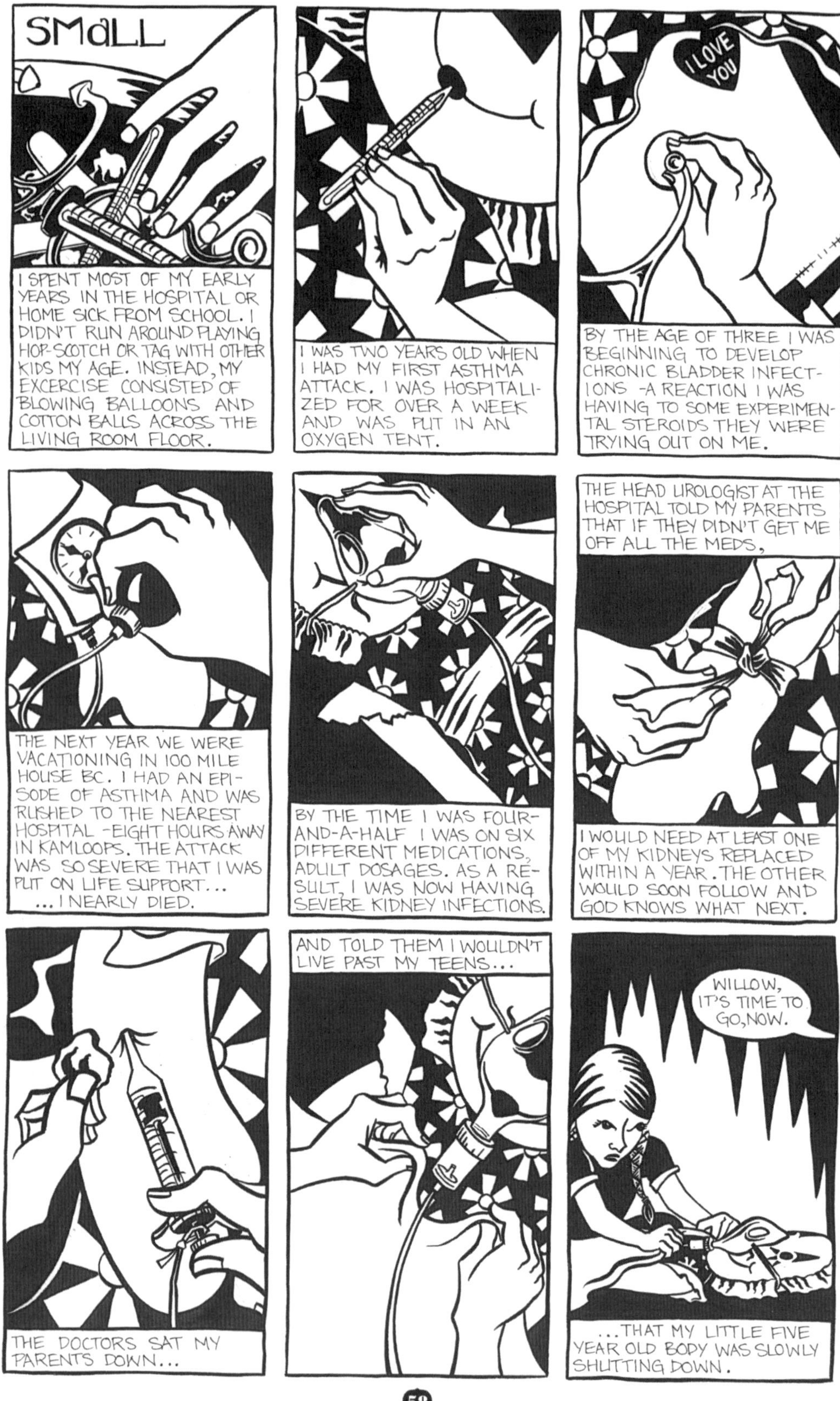
SMALL
I SPENT MOST OF MY EARLY YEARS IN THE HOSPITAL OR HOME SICK FROM SCHOOL. I DIDN'T RUN AROUND PLAYING HOP-SCOTCH OR TAG WITH OTHER KIDS MY AGE. INSTEAD, MY EXCERCISE CONSISTED OF BLOWING BALLOONS AND COTTON BALLS ACROSS THE LIVING ROOM FLOOR.
I WAS TWO YEARS OLD WHEN I HAD MY FIRST ASTHMA ATTACK. I WAS HOSPITALIZED FOR OVER A WEEK AND WAS PUT IN AN OXYGEN TENT.
I LOVE YOU
BY THE AGE OF THREE I WAS BEGINNING TO DEVELOP CHRONIC BLADDER INFECTIONS -A REACTION I WAS HAVING TO SOME EXPERIMENTAL STEROIDS THEY WERE TRYING OUT ON ME.
THE NEXT YEAR WE WERE VACATIONING IN 100 MILE HOUSE BC. I HAD AN EPISODE OF ASTHMA AND WAS RUSHED TO THE NEAREST HOSPITAL -EIGHT HOURS AWAY IN KAMLOOPS. THE ATTACK WAS SO SEVERE THAT I WAS PUT ON LIFE SUPPORT...
...I NEARLY DIED.
BY THE TIME I WAS FOUR-AND-A-HALF I WAS ON SIX DIFFERENT MEDICATIONS, ADULT DOSAGES. AS A RESULT, I WAS NOW HAVING SEVERE KIDNEY INFECTIONS.
THE HEAD UROLOGIST AT THE HOSPITAL TOLD MY PARENTS THAT IF THEY DIDN'T GET ME OFF ALL THE MEDS,
I WOULD NEED AT LEAST ONE OF MY KIDNEYS REPLACED WITHIN A YEAR. THE OTHER WOULD SOON FOLLOW AND GOD KNOWS WHAT NEXT.
THE DOCTORS SAT MY PARENTS DOWN...
AND TOLD THEM I WOULDN'T LIVE PAST MY TEENS...
WILLOW, IT'S TIME TO GO, NOW.
...THAT MY LITTLE FIVE YEAR OLD BODY WAS SLOWLY SHUTTING DOWN.

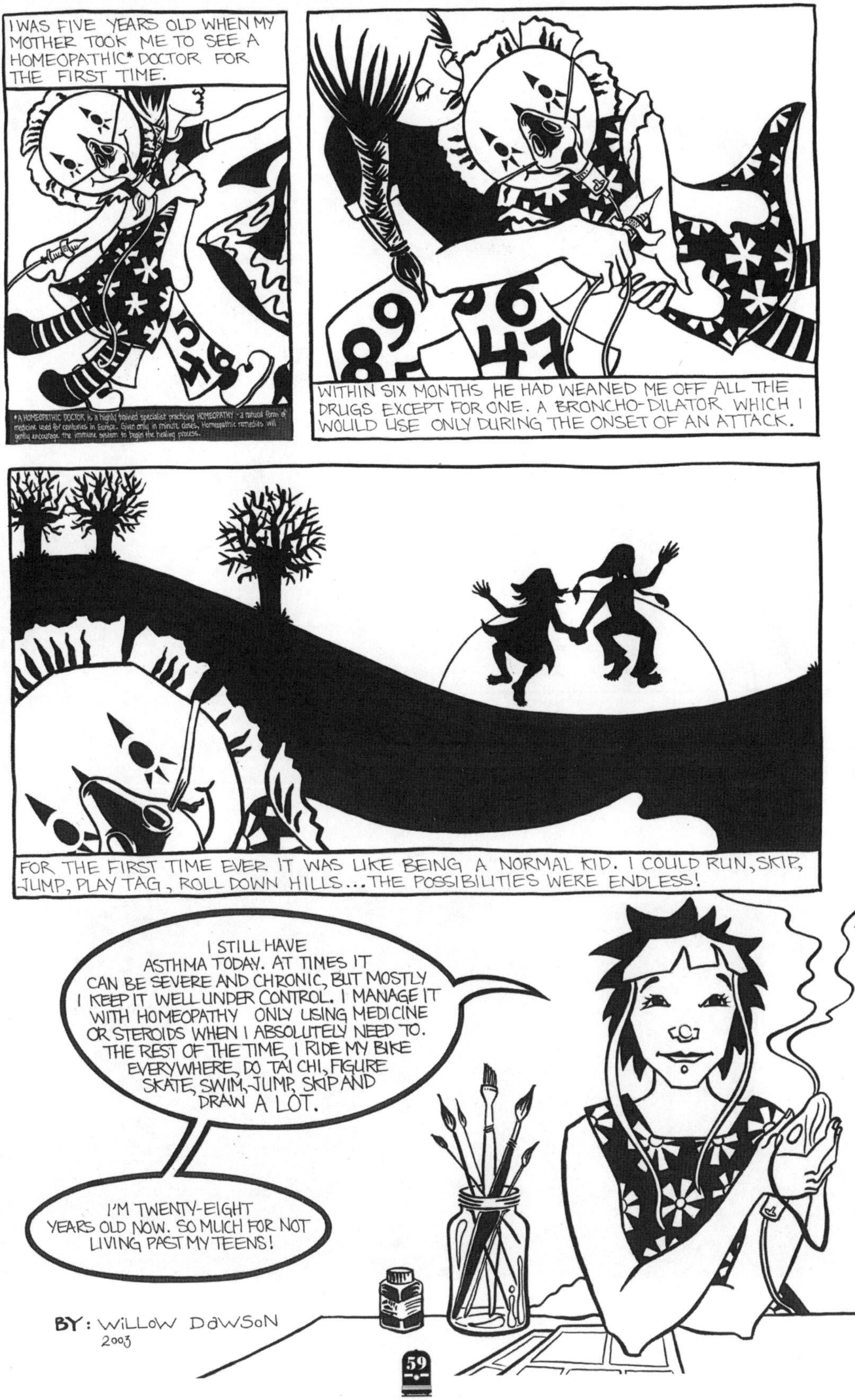
I WAS FIVE YEARS OLD WHEN MY MOTHER TOOK ME TO SEE A HOMEOPATHIC* DOCTOR FOR THE FIRST TIME.
* A HOMEOPATHIC DOCTOR is a highly trained specialist practicing HOMEOPATHY - a natural form of medicine used for centuries in Europe. Given only in minute doses, Homeopathic remedies will gently encourage the immune system to begin the healing process.
WITHIN SIX MONTHS HE HAD WEANED ME OFF ALL THE DRUGS EXCEPT FOR ONE. A BRONCHO-DILATOR WHICH I WOULD USE ONLY DURING THE ONSET OF AN ATTACK.
FOR THE FIRST TIME EVER IT WAS LIKE BEING A NORMAL KID. I COULD RUN, SKIP, JUMP, PLAY TAG, ROLL DOWN HILLS... THE POSSIBILITIES WERE ENDLESS!
I STILL HAVE ASTHMA TODAY. AT TIMES IT CAN BE SEVERE AND CHRONIC, BUT MOSTLY I KEEP IT WELL UNDER CONTROL. I MANAGE IT WITH HOMEOPATHY ONLY USING MEDICINE OR STEROIDS WHEN I ABSOLUTELY NEED TO. THE REST OF THE TIME, I RIDE MY BIKE EVERYWHERE, DO TAI CHI, FIGURE SKATE, SWIM, JUMP, SKIP AND DRAW A LOT.
I'M TWENTY-EIGHT YEARS OLD NOW. SO MUCH FOR NOT LIVING PAST MY TEENS!
BY: WILLOW DAWSON
2003

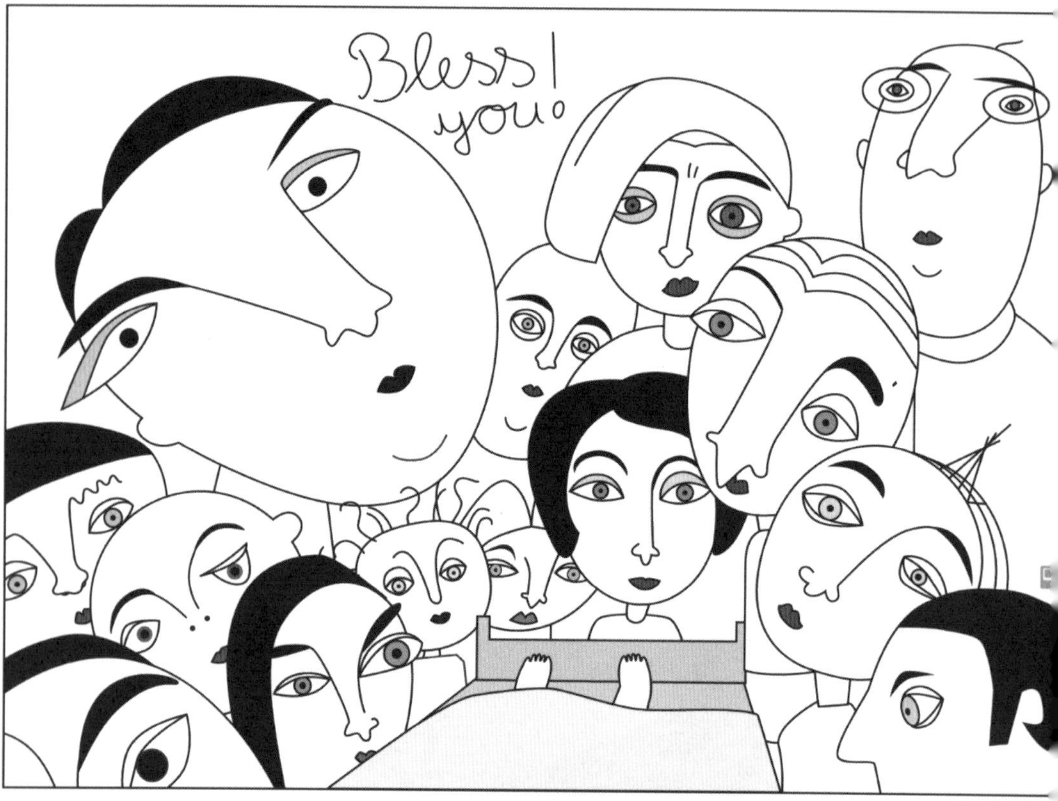
Bless! you!

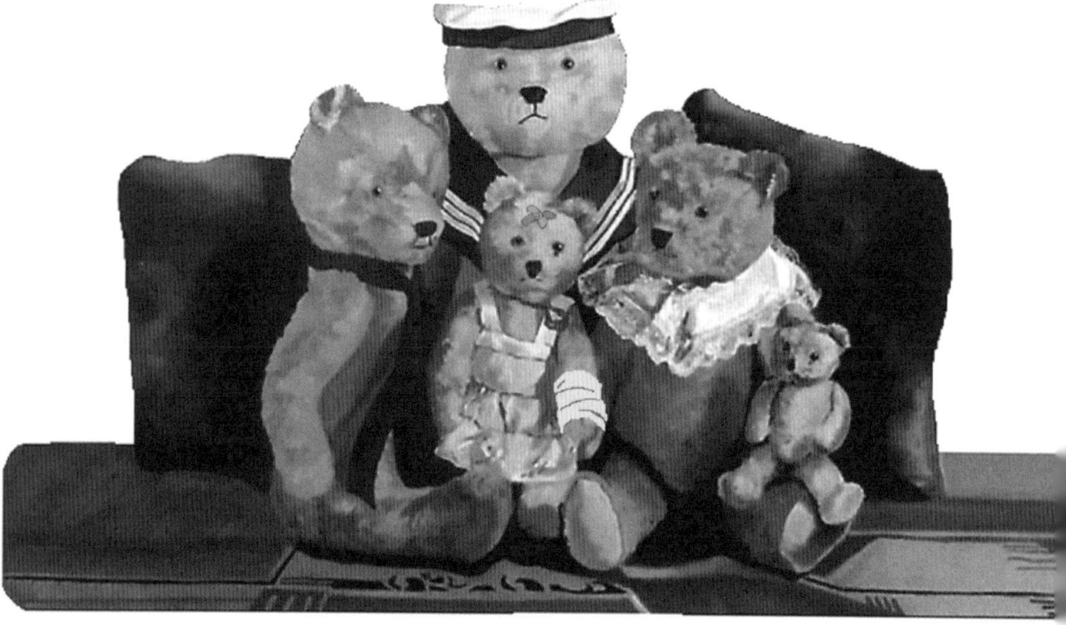

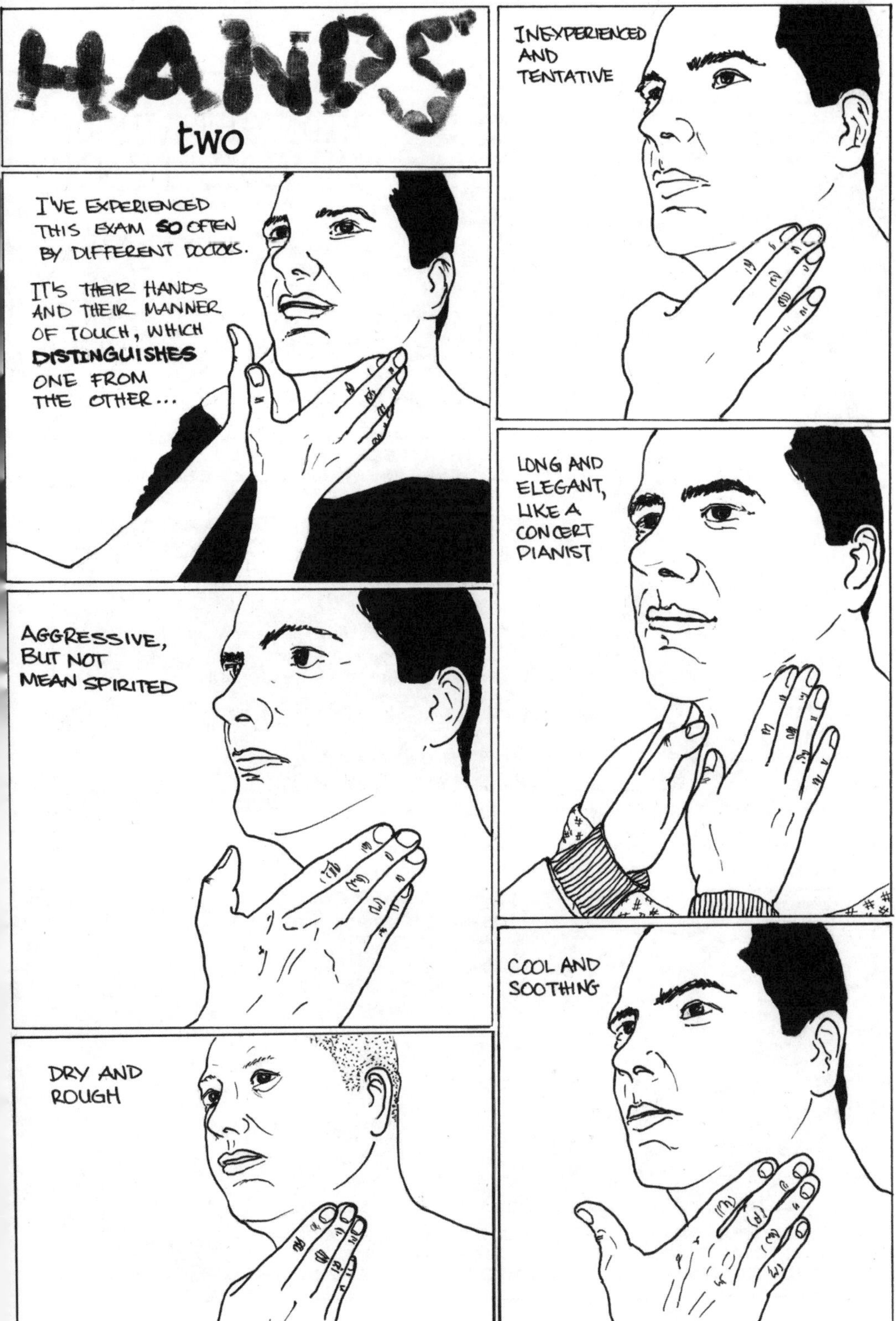
HANDS
two
I'VE EXPERIENCED THIS EXAM SO OFTEN BY DIFFERENT DOCTORS.
IT'S THEIR HANDS AND THEIR MANNER OF TOUCH, WHICH DISTINGUISHES ONE FROM THE OTHER...
INEXPERIENCED AND TENTATIVE
LONG AND ELEGANT, LIKE A CONCERT PIANIST
AGGRESSIVE, BUT NOT MEAN SPIRITED
COOL AND SOOTHING
DRY AND ROUGH
SUKY 03

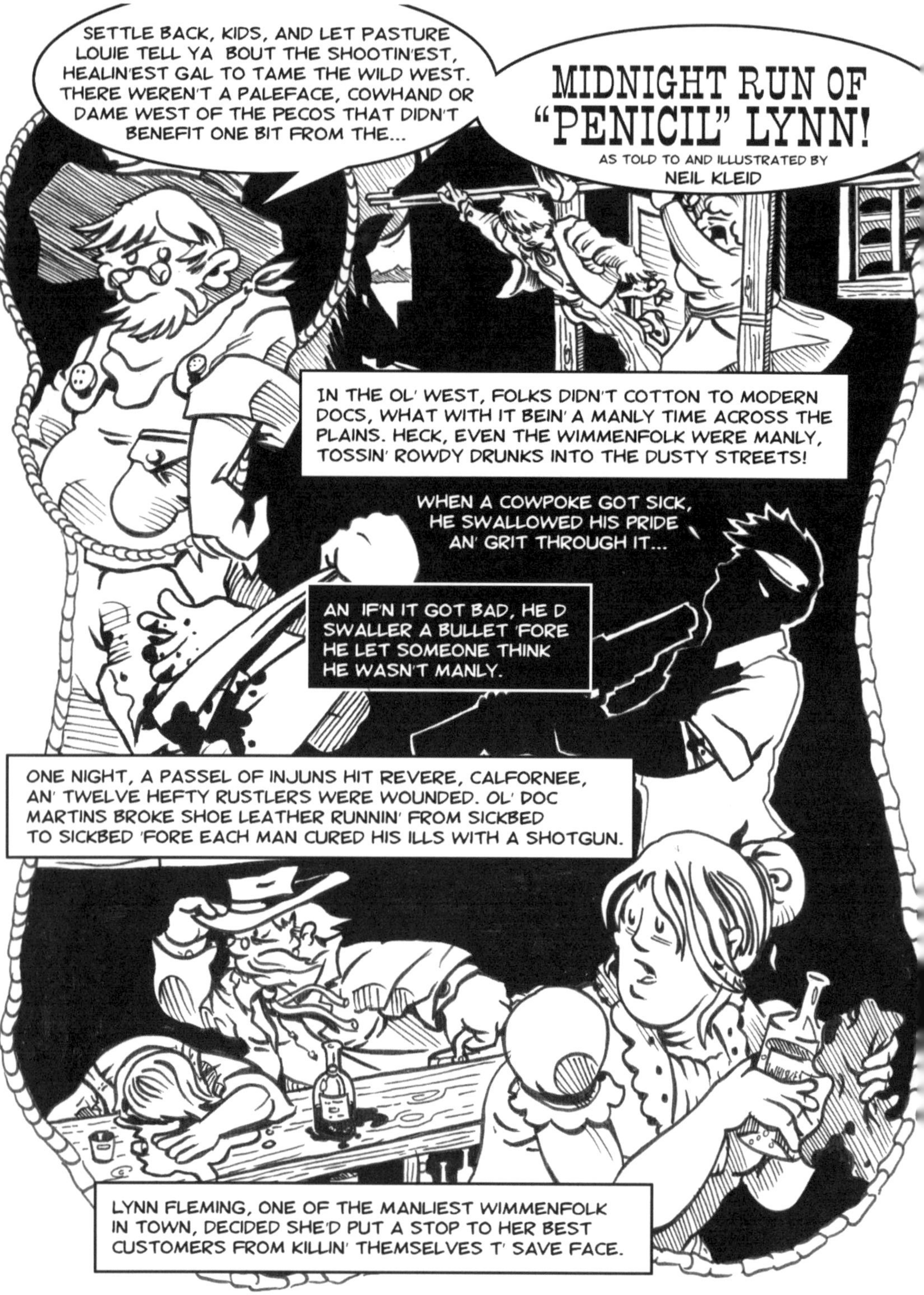
SETTLE BACK, KIDS, AND LET PASTURE LOUIE TELL YA BOUT THE SHOOTIN'EST, HEALIN'EST GAL TO TAME THE WILD WEST. THERE WEREN'T A PALEFACE, COWHAND OR DAME WEST OF THE PECOS THAT DIDN'T BENEFIT ONE BIT FROM THE...
MIDNIGHT RUN OF "PENICIL" LYNN!
AS TOLD TO AND ILLUSTRATED BY
NEIL KLEID
IN THE OL' WEST, FOLKS DIDN'T COTTON TO MODERN DOCS, WHAT WITH IT BEIN' A MANLY TIME ACROSS THE PLAINS. HECK, EVEN THE WIMMENFOLK WERE MANLY, TOSSIN' ROWDY DRUNKS INTO THE DUSTY STREETS!
WHEN A COWPOKE GOT SICK, HE SWALLOWED HIS PRIDE AN' GRIT THROUGH IT...
AN IF'N IT GOT BAD, HE D SWALLER A BULLET 'FORE HE LET SOMEONE THINK HE WASN'T MANLY.
ONE NIGHT, A PASSEL OF INJUNS HIT REVERE, CALFORNEE, AN' TWELVE HEFTY RUSTLERS WERE WOUNDED. OL' DOC MARTINS BROKE SHOE LEATHER RUNNIN' FROM SICKBED TO SICKBED 'FORE EACH MAN CURED HIS ILLS WITH A SHOTGUN.
LYNN FLEMING, ONE OF THE MANLIEST WIMMENFOLK IN TOWN, DECIDED SHE'D PUT A STOP TO HER BEST CUSTOMERS FROM KILLIN' THEMSELVES T' SAVE FACE.

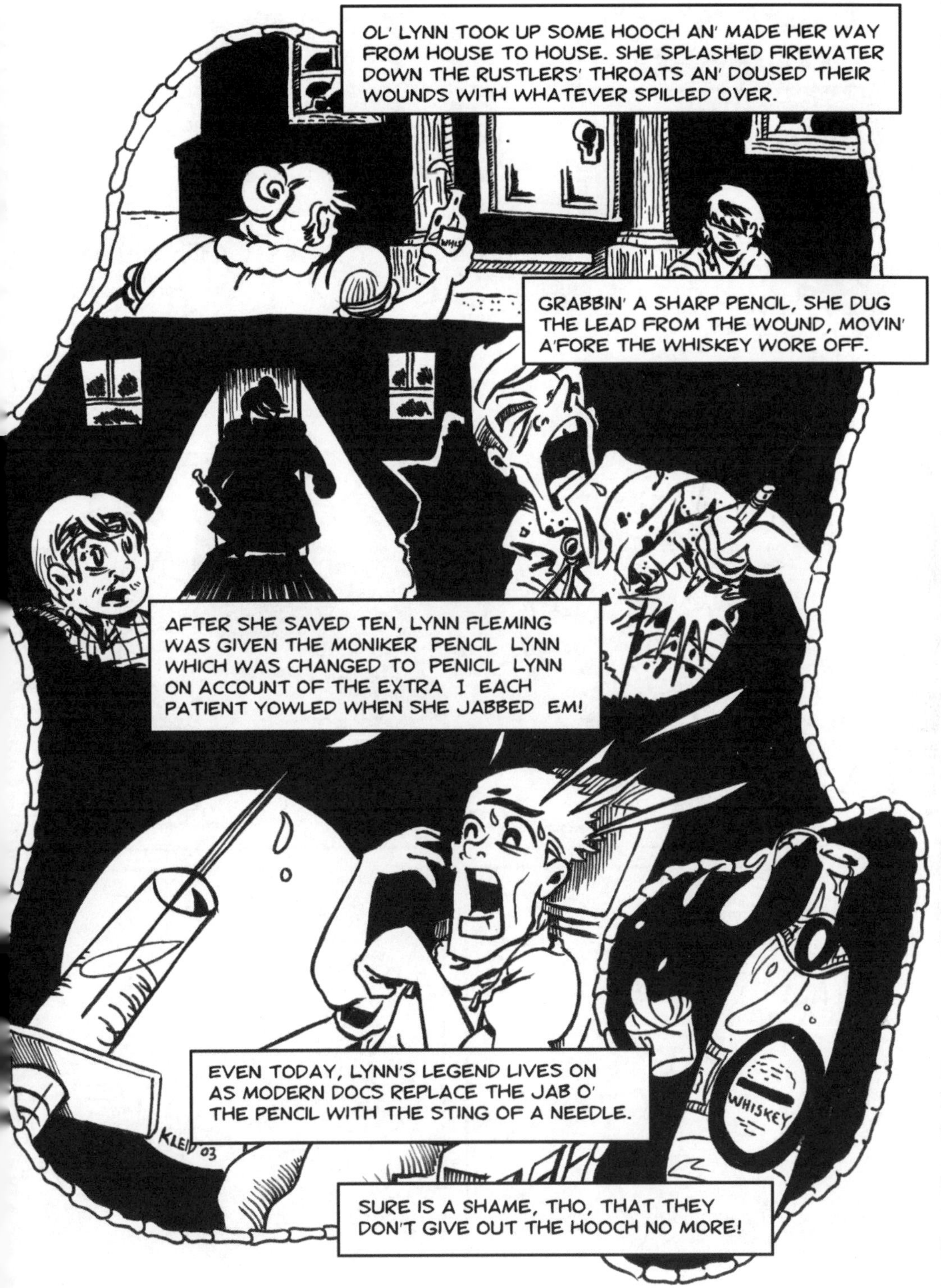
OL' LYNN TOOK UP SOME HOOCH AN' MADE HER WAY FROM HOUSE TO HOUSE. SHE SPLASHED FIREWATER DOWN THE RUSTLERS' THROATS AN' DOUSED THEIR WOUNDS WITH WHATEVER SPILLED OVER.
GRABBIN' A SHARP PENCIL, SHE DUG THE LEAD FROM THE WOUND, MOVIN' A'FORE THE WHISKEY WORE OFF.
AFTER SHE SAVED TEN, LYNN FLEMING WAS GIVEN THE MONIKER PENCIL LYNN WHICH WAS CHANGED TO PENICIL LYNN ON ACCOUNT OF THE EXTRA I EACH PATIENT YOWLED WHEN SHE JABBED EM!
EVEN TODAY, LYNN'S LEGEND LIVES ON AS MODERN DOCS REPLACE THE JAB O' THE PENCIL WITH THE STING OF A NEEDLE.
WHISKEY
KLEID 03
SURE IS A SHAME, THO, THAT THEY DON'T GIVE OUT THE HOOCH NO MORE!

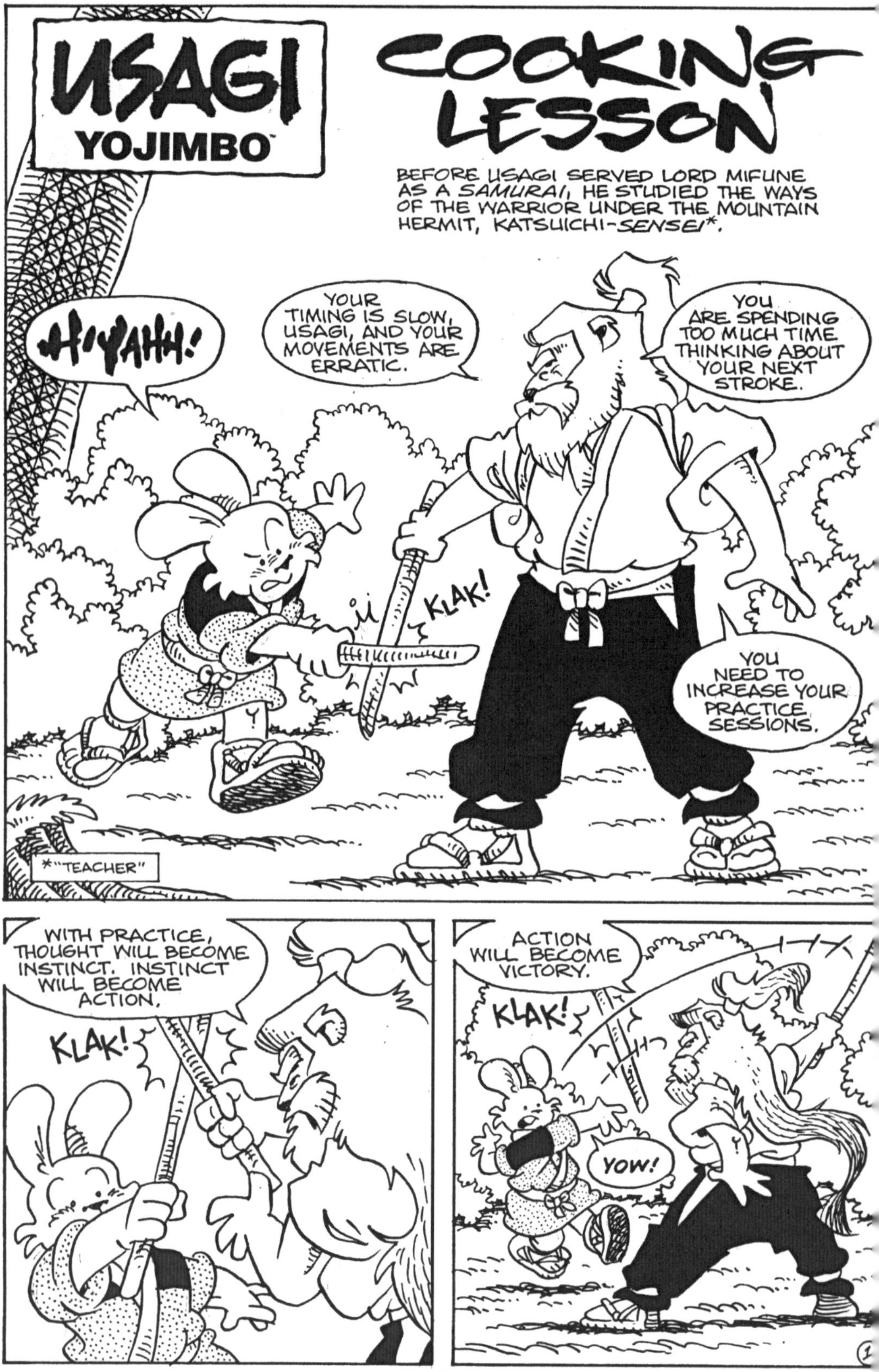
USAGI YOJIMBO
COOKING LESSON
BEFORE USAGI SERVED LORD MIFUNE AS A *SAMURAI*, HE STUDIED THE WAYS OF THE WARRIOR UNDER THE MOUNTAIN HERMIT, KATSUICHI-*SENSEI**.
HI-YAHH!
YOUR TIMING IS SLOW, USAGI, AND YOUR MOVEMENTS ARE ERRATIC.
YOU ARE SPENDING TOO MUCH TIME THINKING ABOUT YOUR NEXT STROKE.
KLAK!
YOU NEED TO INCREASE YOUR PRACTICE SESSIONS.
*"TEACHER"
WITH PRACTICE, THOUGHT WILL BECOME INSTINCT. INSTINCT WILL BECOME ACTION.
KLAK!
ACTION WILL BECOME VICTORY.
KLAK!
YOW!

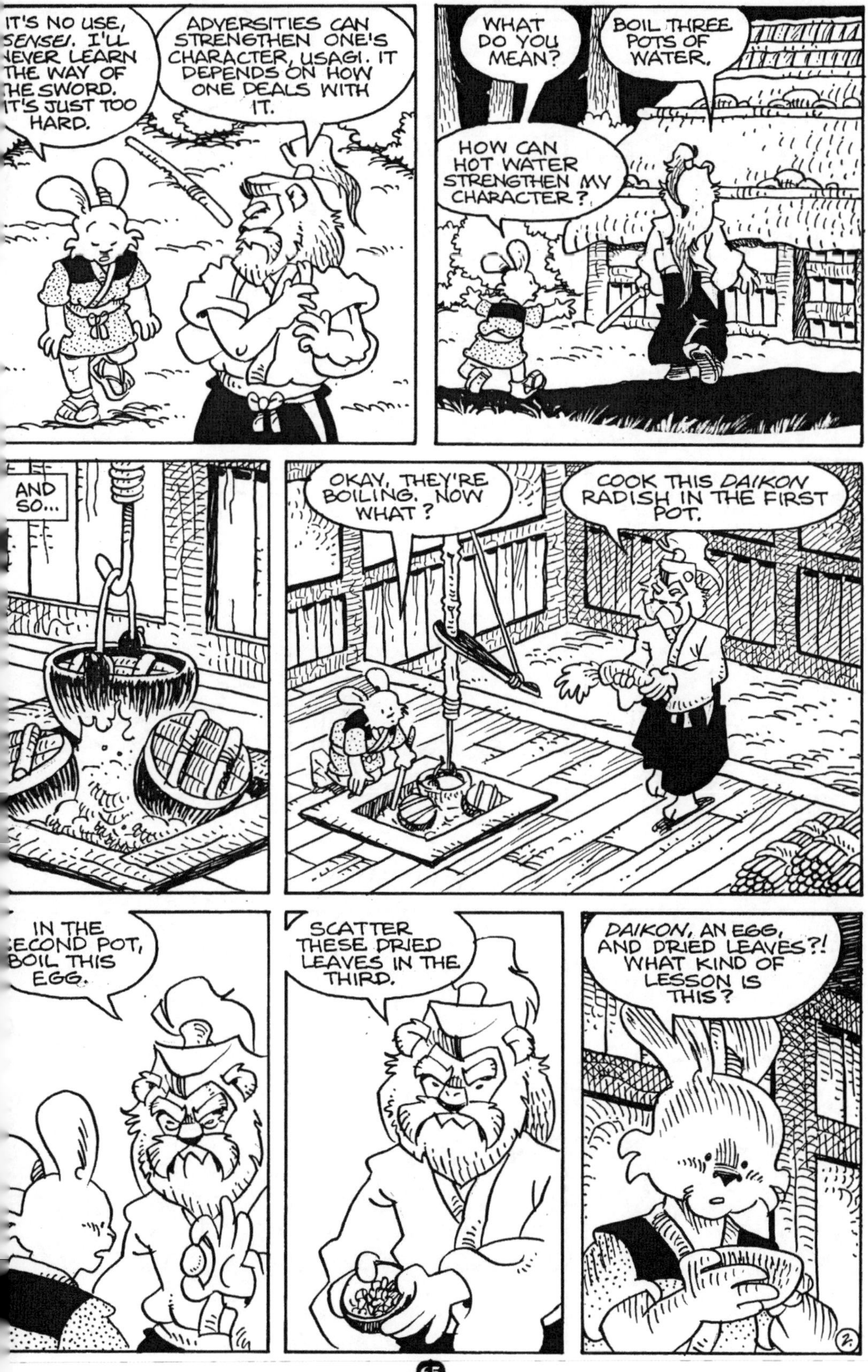
IT'S NO USE, SENSEI. I'LL NEVER LEARN THE WAY OF THE SWORD. IT'S JUST TOO HARD.
ADVERSITIES CAN STRENGTHEN ONE'S CHARACTER, USAGI. IT DEPENDS ON HOW ONE DEALS WITH IT.
WHAT DO YOU MEAN?
BOIL THREE POTS OF WATER.
HOW CAN HOT WATER STRENGTHEN MY CHARACTER?
AND SO...
OKAY, THEY'RE BOILING. NOW WHAT?
COOK THIS DAIKON RADISH IN THE FIRST POT.
IN THE SECOND POT, BOIL THIS EGG.
SCATTER THESE DRIED LEAVES IN THE THIRD.
DAIKON, AN EGG, AND DRIED LEAVES?! WHAT KIND OF LESSON IS THIS?
2.

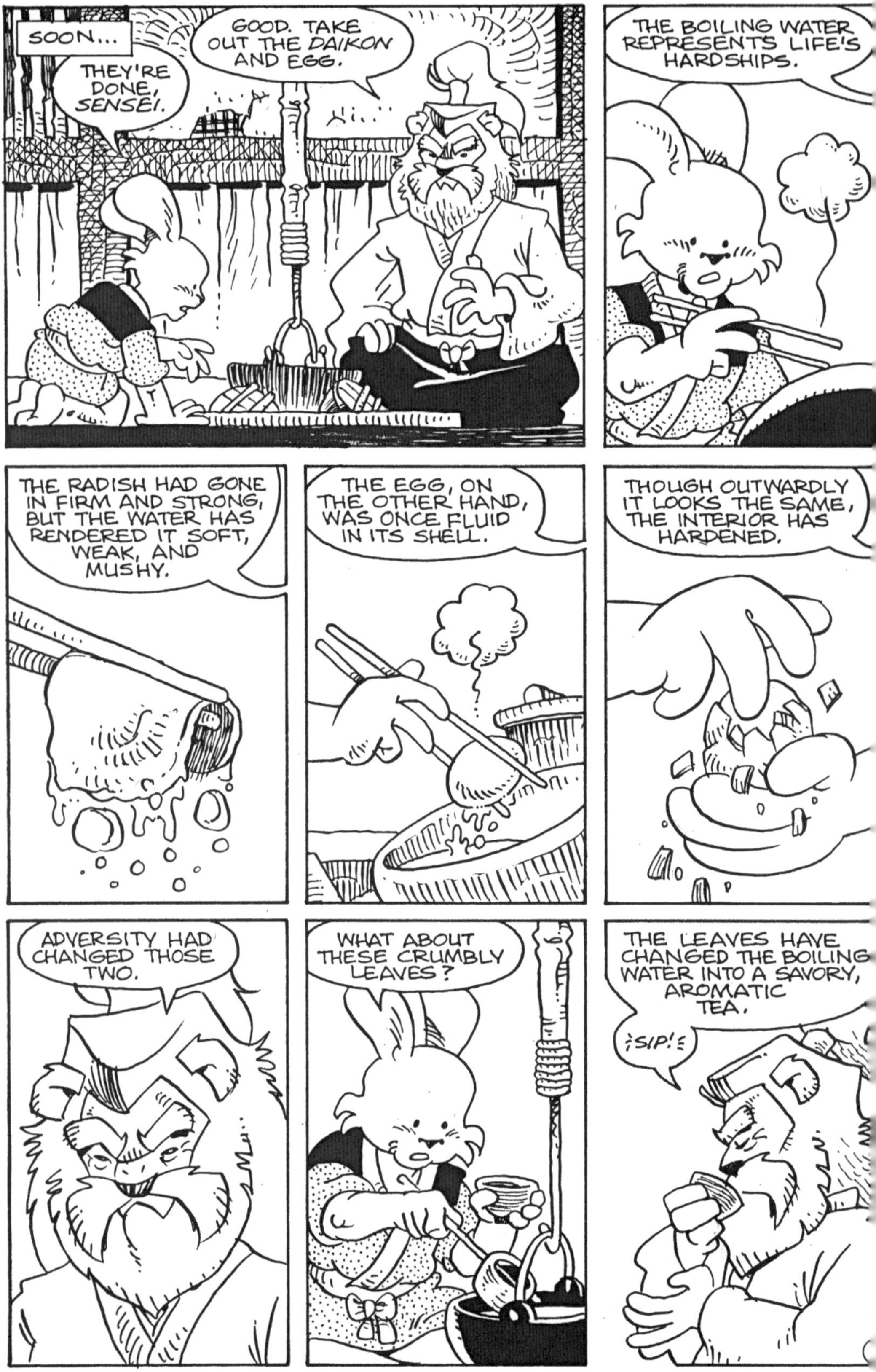
SOON...
THEY'RE DONE, *SENSEI*.
GOOD. TAKE OUT THE *DAIKON* AND EGG.
THE BOILING WATER REPRESENTS LIFE'S HARDSHIPS.
THE RADISH HAD GONE IN FIRM AND STRONG, BUT THE WATER HAS RENDERED IT SOFT, WEAK, AND MUSHY.
THE EGG, ON THE OTHER HAND, WAS ONCE FLUID IN ITS SHELL.
THOUGH OUTWARDLY IT LOOKS THE SAME, THE INTERIOR HAS HARDENED.
ADVERSITY HAD CHANGED THOSE TWO.
WHAT ABOUT THESE CRUMBLY LEAVES?
THE LEAVES HAVE CHANGED THE BOILING WATER INTO A SAVORY, AROMATIC TEA.
SIP!

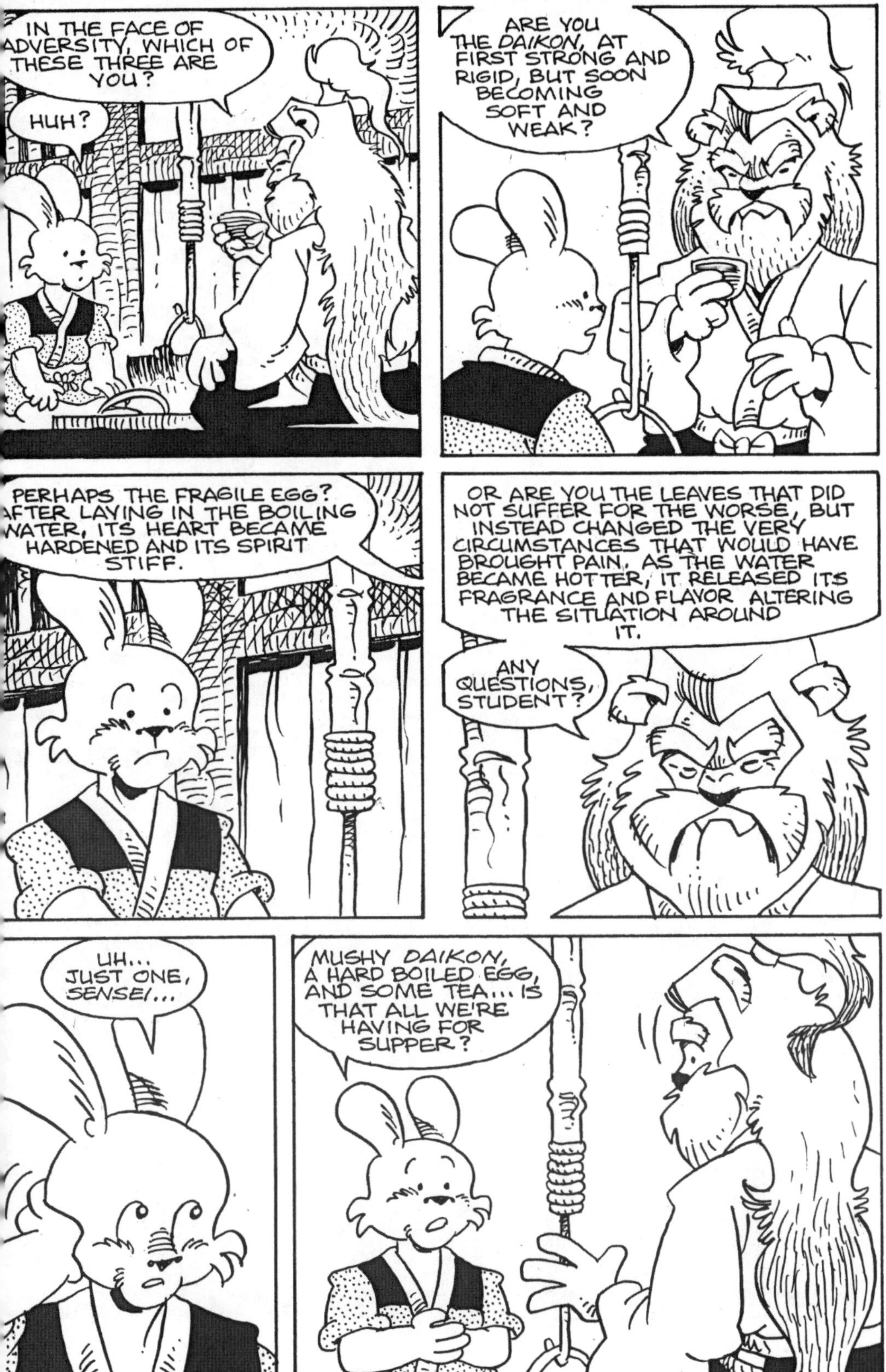
IN THE FACE OF ADVERSITY, WHICH OF THESE THREE ARE YOU?
HUH?
ARE YOU THE *DAIKON*, AT FIRST STRONG AND RIGID, BUT SOON BECOMING SOFT AND WEAK?
PERHAPS THE FRAGILE EGG? AFTER LAYING IN THE BOILING WATER, ITS HEART BECAME HARDENED AND ITS SPIRIT STIFF.
OR ARE YOU THE LEAVES THAT DID NOT SUFFER FOR THE WORSE, BUT INSTEAD CHANGED THE VERY CIRCUMSTANCES THAT WOULD HAVE BROUGHT PAIN. AS THE WATER BECAME HOTTER, IT RELEASED ITS FRAGRANCE AND FLAVOR ALTERING THE SITUATION AROUND IT.
ANY QUESTIONS, STUDENT?
UH... JUST ONE, *SENSEI*...
MUSHY *DAIKON*, A HARD BOILED EGG, AND SOME TEA... IS THAT ALL WE'RE HAVING FOR SUPPER?

THE END.

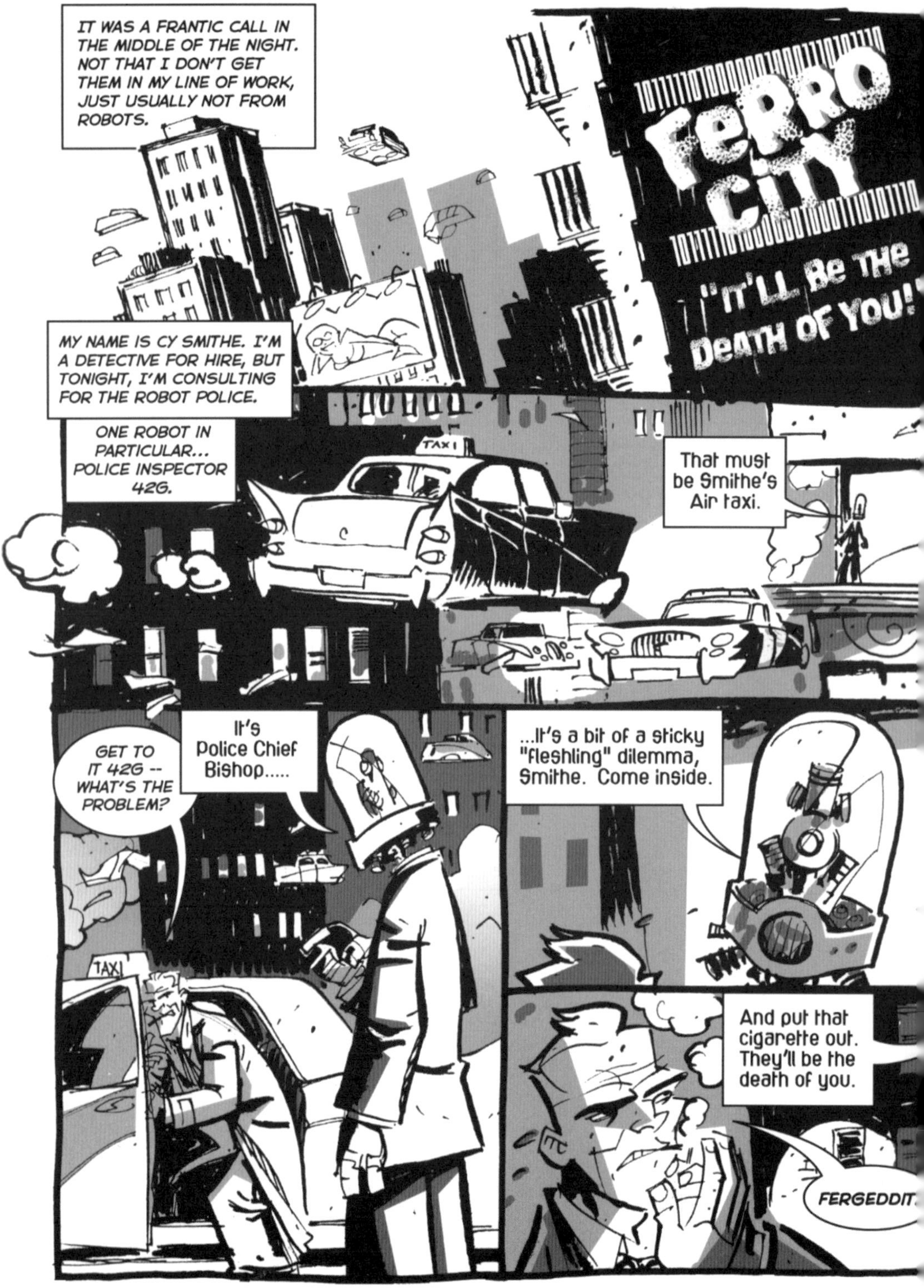

Ferro City created by Jason Armstrong

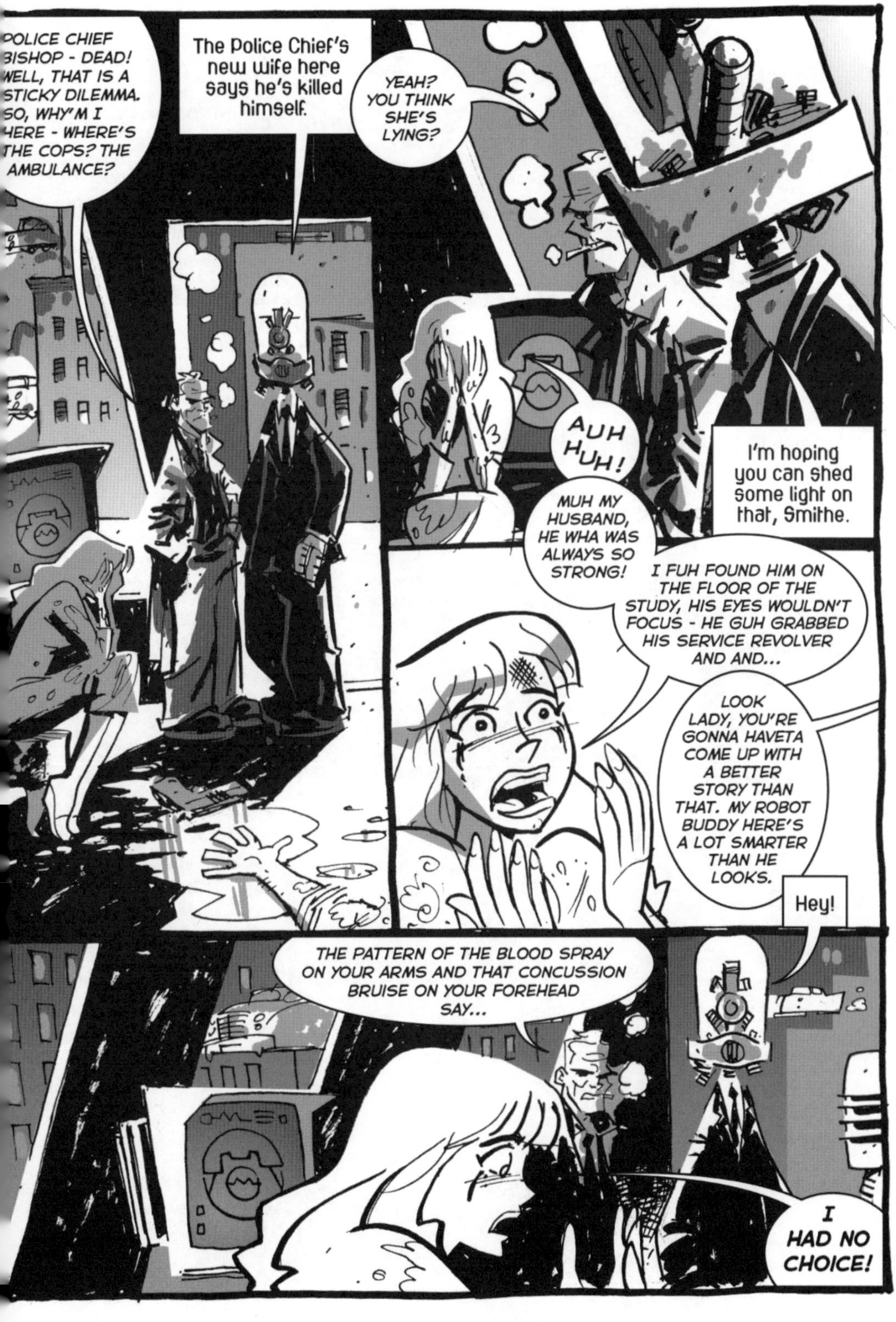
POLICE CHIEF BISHOP - DEAD! WELL, THAT IS A STICKY DILEMMA. SO, WHY'M I HERE - WHERE'S THE COPS? THE AMBULANCE?
The Police Chief's new wife here says he's killed himself.
YEAH? YOU THINK SHE'S LYING?
AUH HUH!
I'm hoping you can shed some light on that, Smithe.
MUH MY HUSBAND, HE WHA WAS ALWAYS SO STRONG!
I FUH FOUND HIM ON THE FLOOR OF THE STUDY, HIS EYES WOULDN'T FOCUS - HE GUH GRABBED HIS SERVICE REVOLVER AND AND...
LOOK LADY, YOU'RE GONNA HAVETA COME UP WITH A BETTER STORY THAN THAT. MY ROBOT BUDDY HERE'S A LOT SMARTER THAN HE LOOKS.
Hey!
THE PATTERN OF THE BLOOD SPRAY ON YOUR ARMS AND THAT CONCUSSION BRUISE ON YOUR FOREHEAD SAY...
I HAD NO CHOICE!

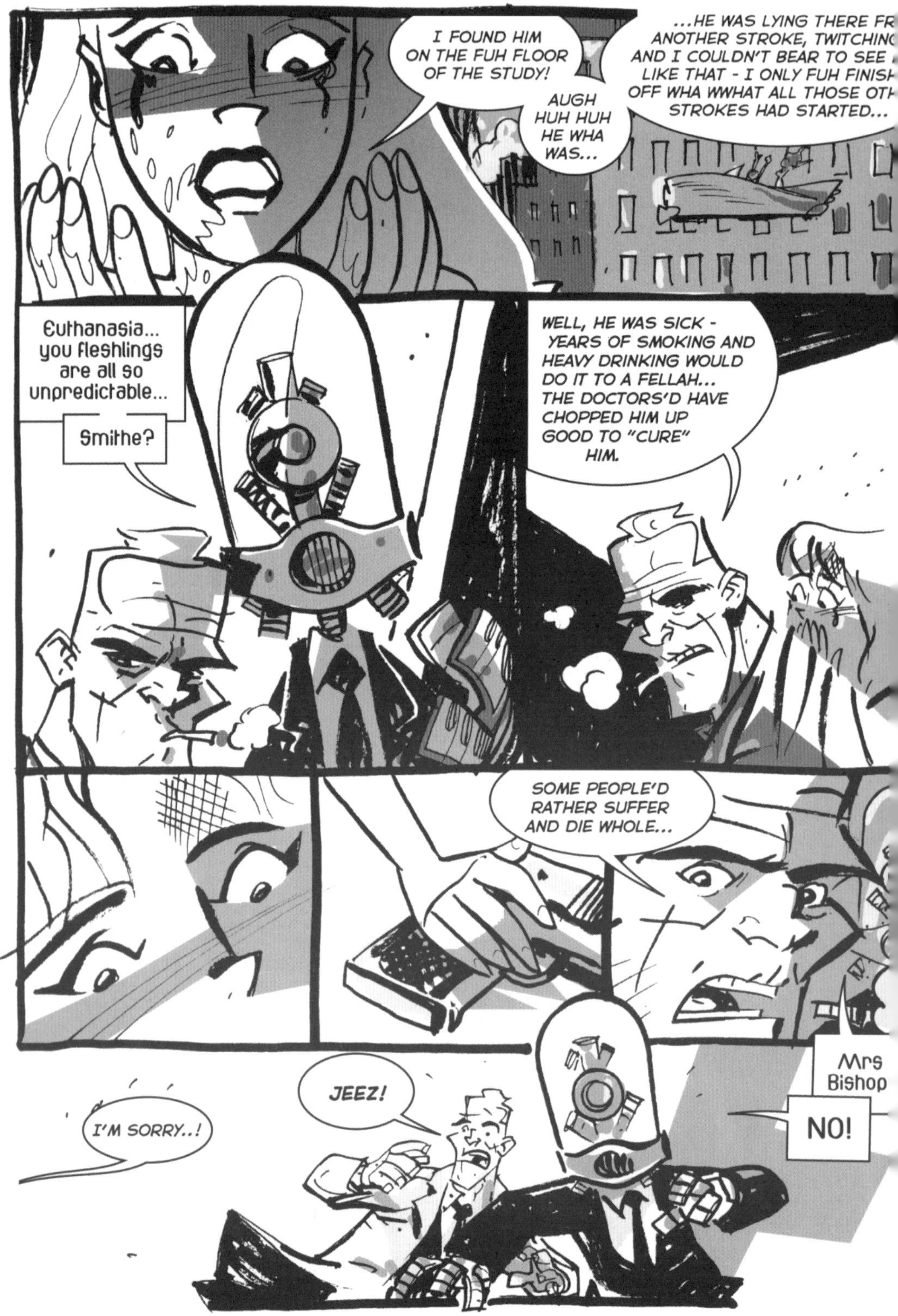
I FOUND HIM ON THE FUH FLOOR OF THE STUDY!
AUGH HUH HUH HE WHA WAS...
...HE WAS LYING THERE FR ANOTHER STROKE, TWITCHIN AND I COULDN'T BEAR TO SEE LIKE THAT - I ONLY FUH FINIS OFF WHA WWHAT ALL THOSE OT STROKES HAD STARTED...
Euthanasia... you fleshlings are all so unpredictable...
Smithe?
WELL, HE WAS SICK - YEARS OF SMOKING AND HEAVY DRINKING WOULD DO IT TO A FELLAH... THE DOCTORS'D HAVE CHOPPED HIM UP GOOD TO "CURE" HIM.
SOME PEOPLE'D RATHER SUFFER AND DIE WHOLE...
Mrs Bishop
NO!
JEEZ!
I'M SORRY..!

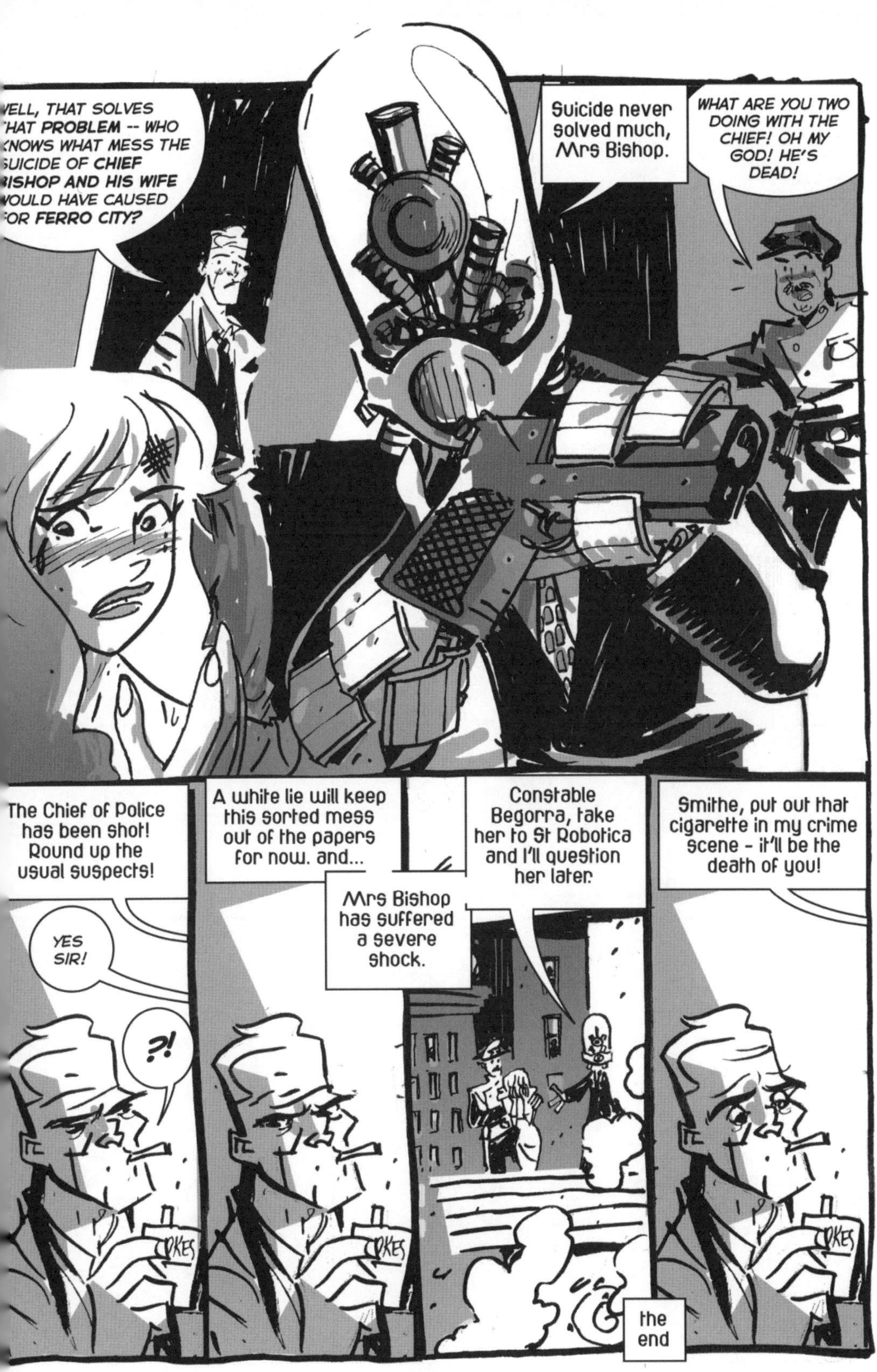
WELL, THAT SOLVES THAT PROBLEM -- WHO KNOWS WHAT MESS THE SUICIDE OF CHIEF BISHOP AND HIS WIFE WOULD HAVE CAUSED FOR FERRO CITY?
Suicide never solved much, Mrs Bishop.
WHAT ARE YOU TWO DOING WITH THE CHIEF! OH MY GOD! HE'S DEAD!
The Chief of Police has been shot! Round up the usual suspects!
YES SIR!
?!
COKES
A white lie will keep this sorted mess out of the papers for now. and...
Mrs Bishop has suffered a severe shock.
COKES
Constable Begorra, take her to St Robotica and I'll question her later.
Smithe, put out that cigarette in my crime scene - it'll be the death of you!
COKES
the end

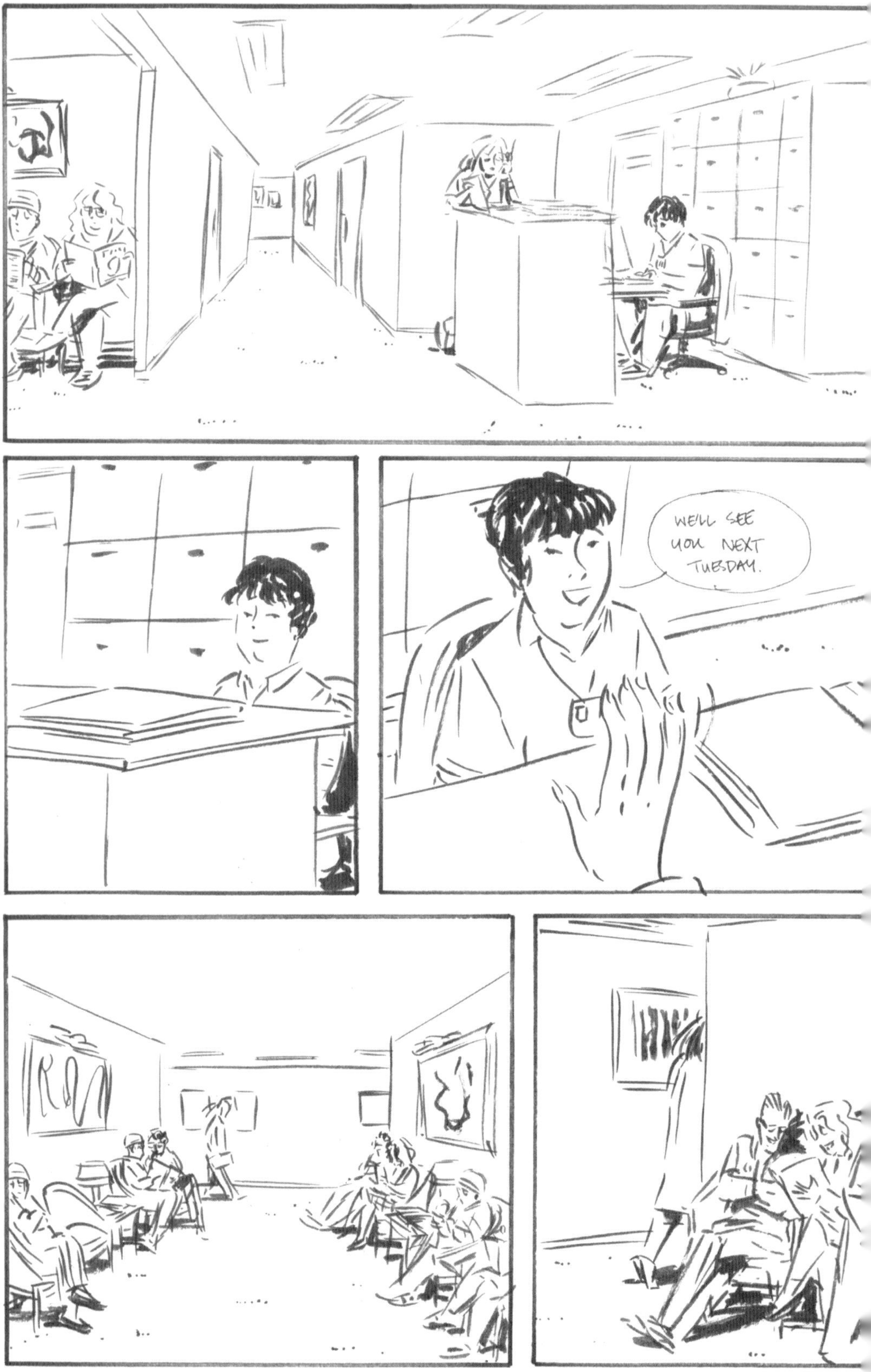
WE'LL SEE YOU NEXT TUESDAY.

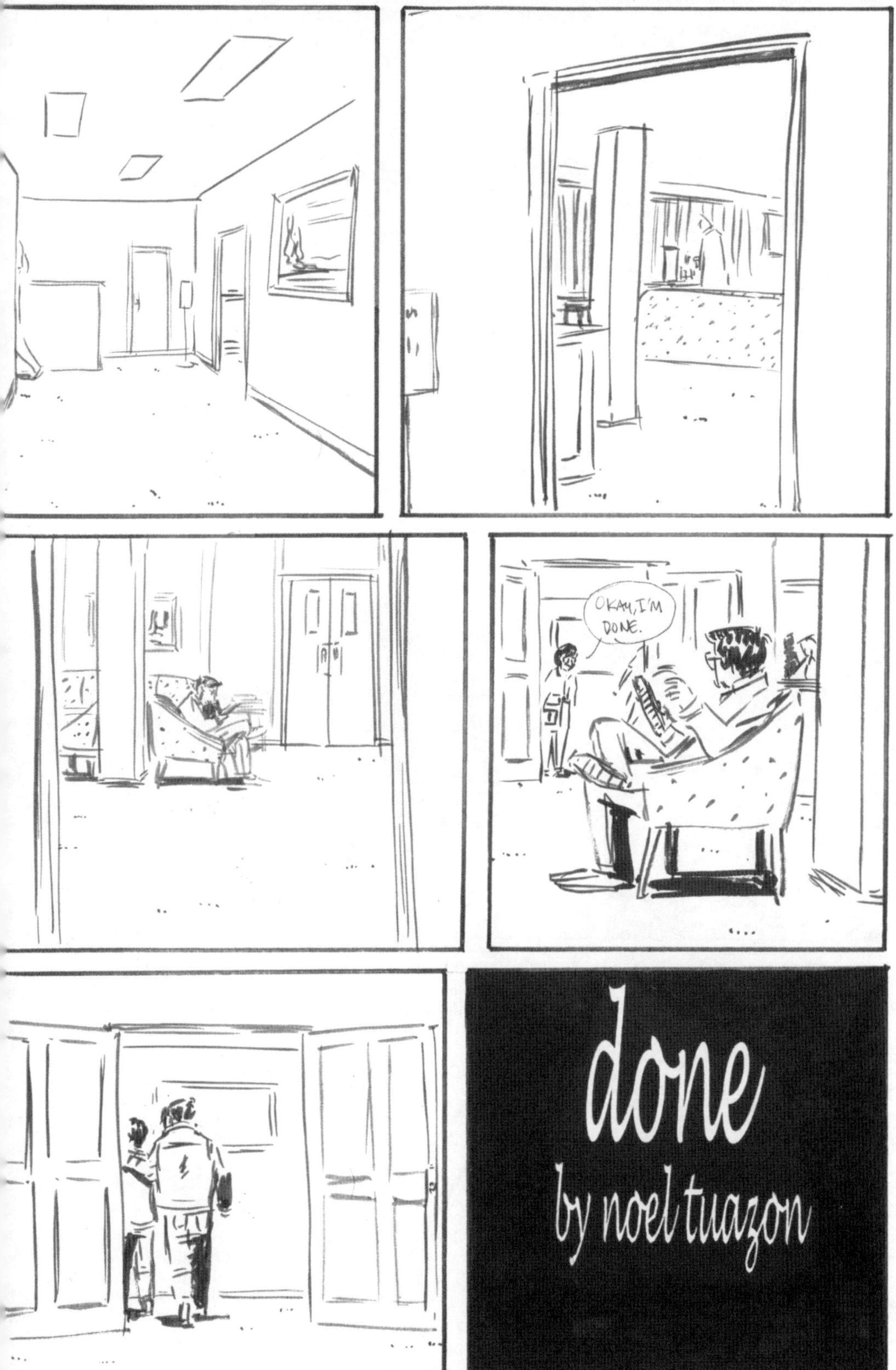

done

by noel tuazon

PERSIMMONS

the last days of norman bethune

WORDS:
DEREK BROWN

PICTURES:
DOMINIC BUGATTO

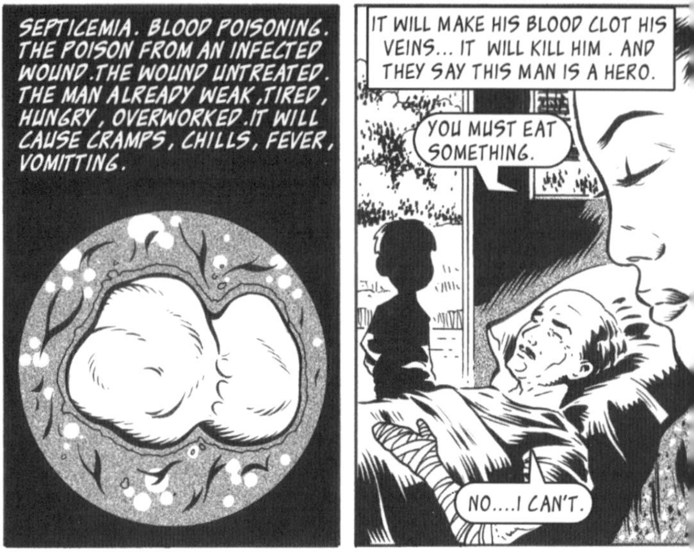

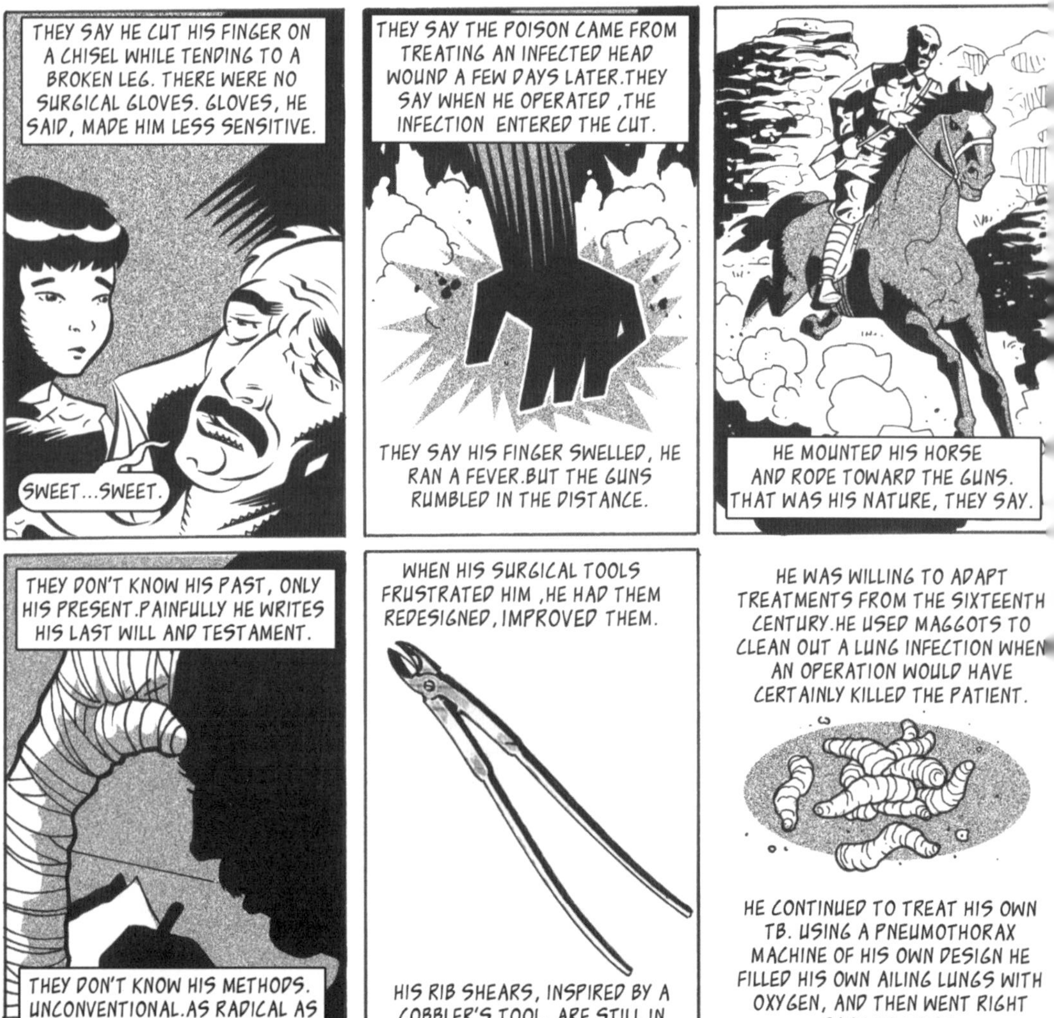

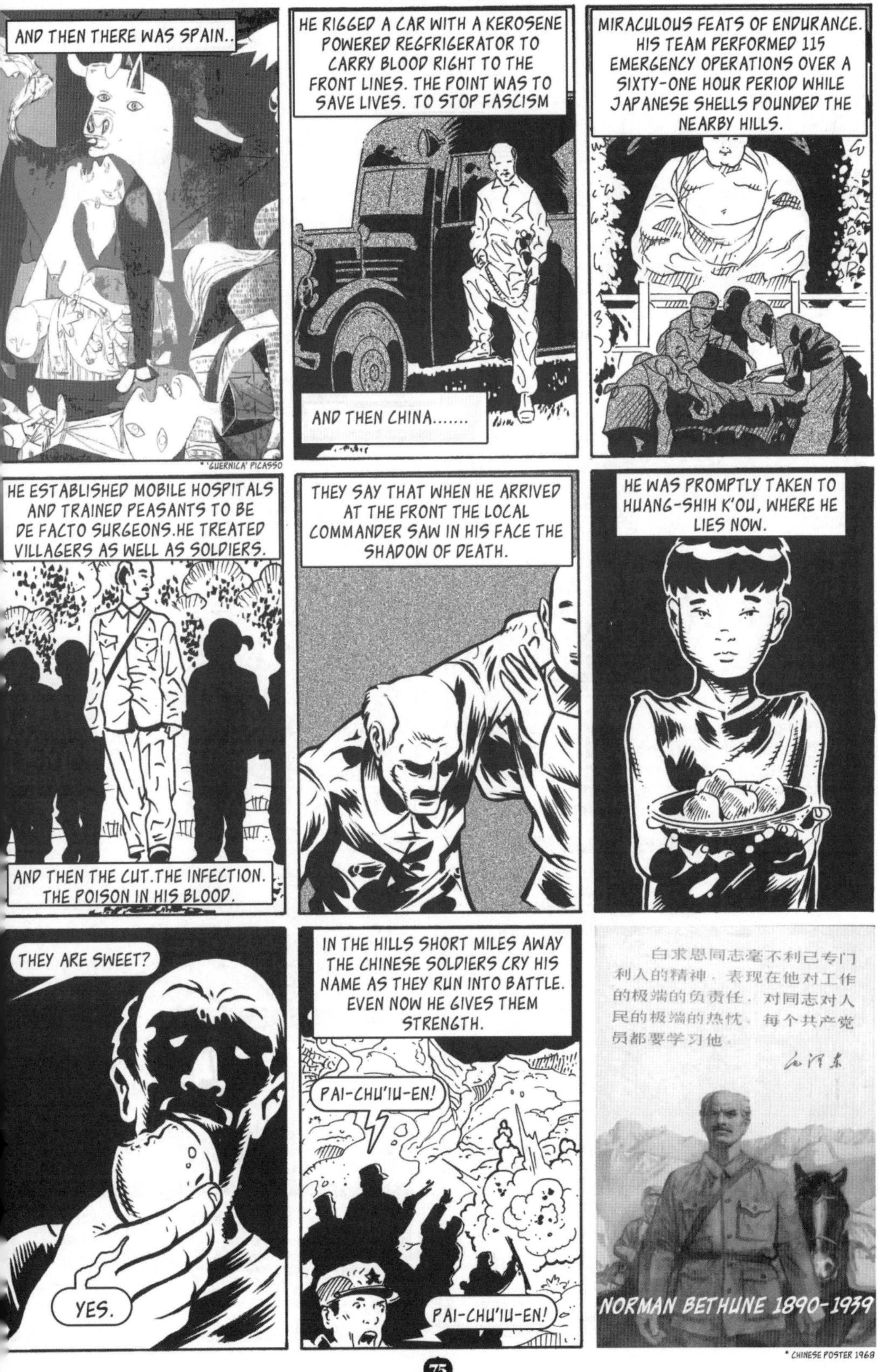

* 'GUERNICA' PICASSO

* CHINESE POSTER 1968

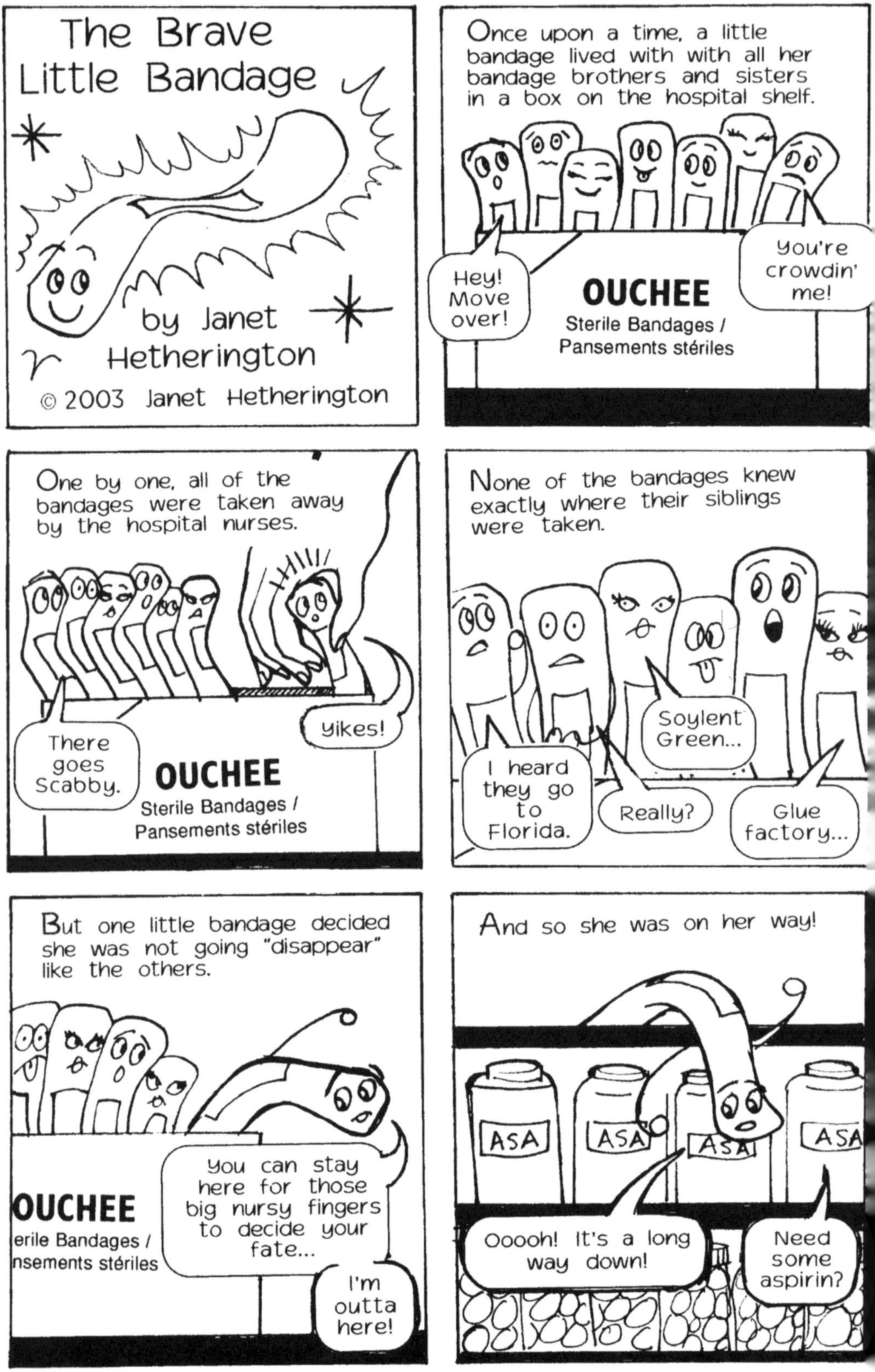

The Brave Little Bandage
by Janet Hetherington
© 2003 Janet Hetherington
Once upon a time, a little bandage lived with with all her bandage brothers and sisters in a box on the hospital shelf.
Hey! Move over!
OUCHEE
Sterile Bandages / Pansements stériles
You're crowdin' me!
One by one, all of the bandages were taken away by the hospital nurses.
There goes Scabby.
OUCHEE
Sterile Bandages / Pansements stériles
Yikes!
None of the bandages knew exactly where their siblings were taken.
I heard they go to Florida.
Really?
Soylent Green...
Glue factory...
But one little bandage decided she was not going "disappear" like the others.
OUCHEE
erile Bandages / nsements stériles
You can stay here for those big nursy fingers to decide your fate...
I'm outta here!
And so she was on her way!
ASA
ASA
ASA
ASA
Ooooh! It's a long way down!
Need some aspirin?

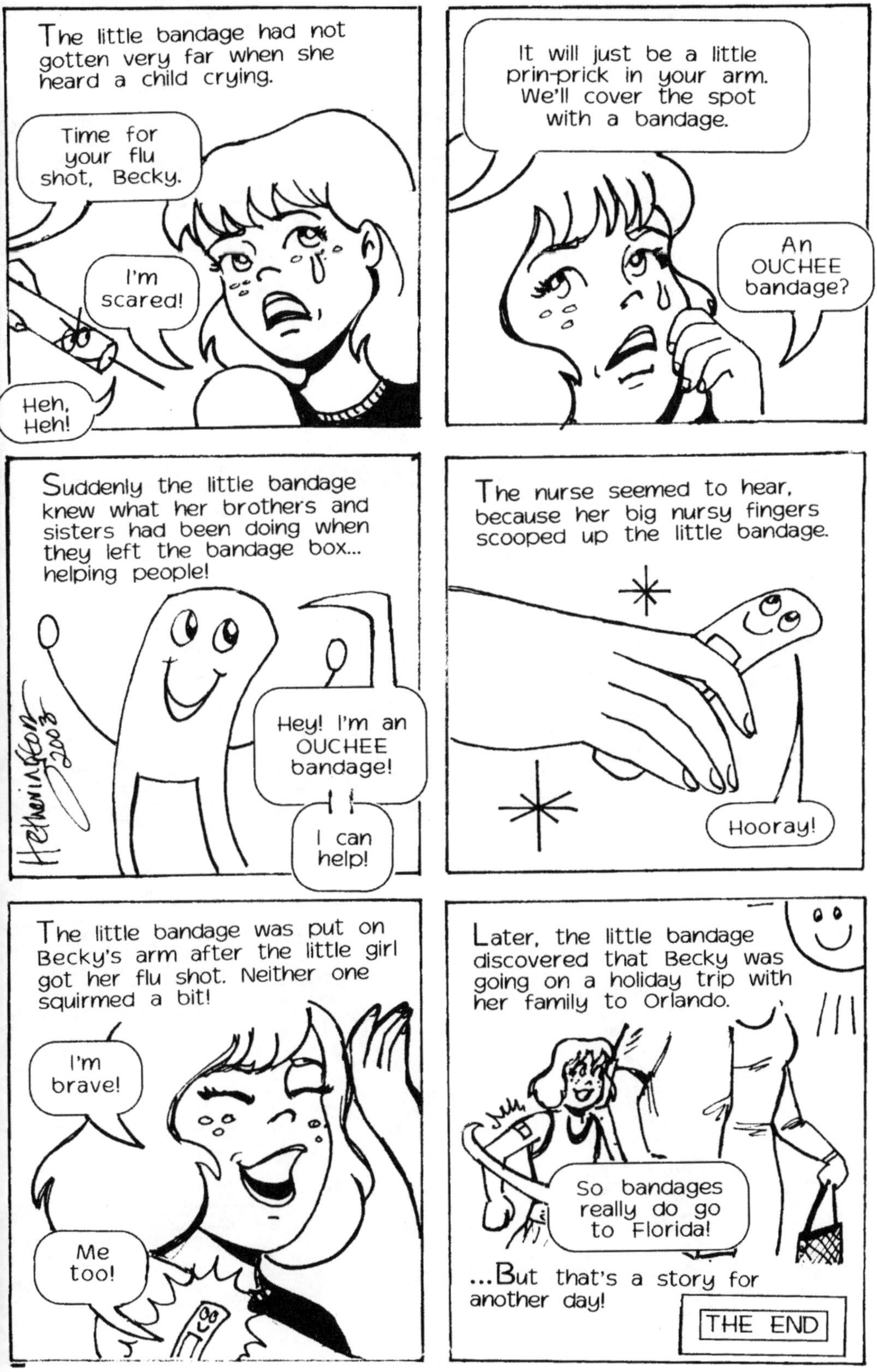
The little bandage had not gotten very far when she heard a child crying.
Time for your flu shot, Becky.
I'm scared!
Heh, Heh!
It will just be a little prin-prick in your arm. We'll cover the spot with a bandage.
An OUCHEE bandage?
Suddenly the little bandage knew what her brothers and sisters had been doing when they left the bandage box... helping people!
Hey! I'm an OUCHEE bandage!
I can help!
The nurse seemed to hear, because her big nursy fingers scooped up the little bandage.
Hooray!
The little bandage was put on Becky's arm after the little girl got her flu shot. Neither one squirmed a bit!
I'm brave!
Me too!
Later, the little bandage discovered that Becky was going on a holiday trip with her family to Orlando.
So bandages really do go to Florida!
...But that's a story for another day!
THE END

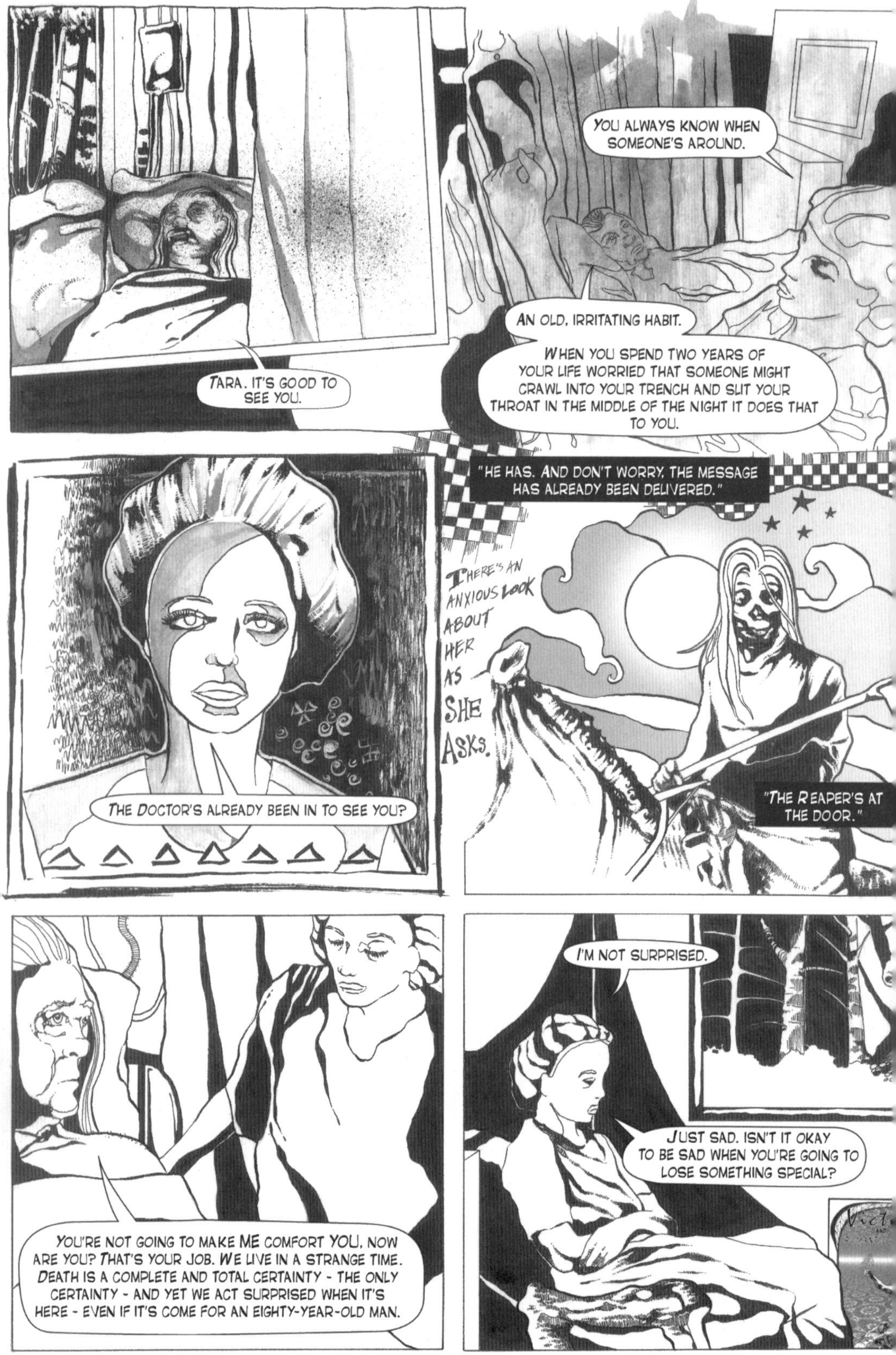
TARA. IT'S GOOD TO SEE YOU.
YOU ALWAYS KNOW WHEN SOMEONE'S AROUND.
AN OLD, IRRITATING HABIT.
WHEN YOU SPEND TWO YEARS OF YOUR LIFE WORRIED THAT SOMEONE MIGHT CRAWL INTO YOUR TRENCH AND SLIT YOUR THROAT IN THE MIDDLE OF THE NIGHT IT DOES THAT TO YOU.
THE DOCTOR'S ALREADY BEEN IN TO SEE YOU?
"HE HAS. AND DON'T WORRY, THE MESSAGE HAS ALREADY BEEN DELIVERED."
THERE'S AN ANXIOUS LOOK ABOUT HER AS SHE ASKS.
"THE REAPER'S AT THE DOOR."
YOU'RE NOT GOING TO MAKE ME COMFORT YOU, NOW ARE YOU? THAT'S YOUR JOB. WE LIVE IN A STRANGE TIME. DEATH IS A COMPLETE AND TOTAL CERTAINTY - THE ONLY CERTAINTY - AND YET WE ACT SURPRISED WHEN IT'S HERE - EVEN IF IT'S COME FOR AN EIGHTY-YEAR-OLD MAN.
I'M NOT SURPRISED.
JUST SAD. ISN'T IT OKAY TO BE SAD WHEN YOU'RE GOING TO LOSE SOMETHING SPECIAL?

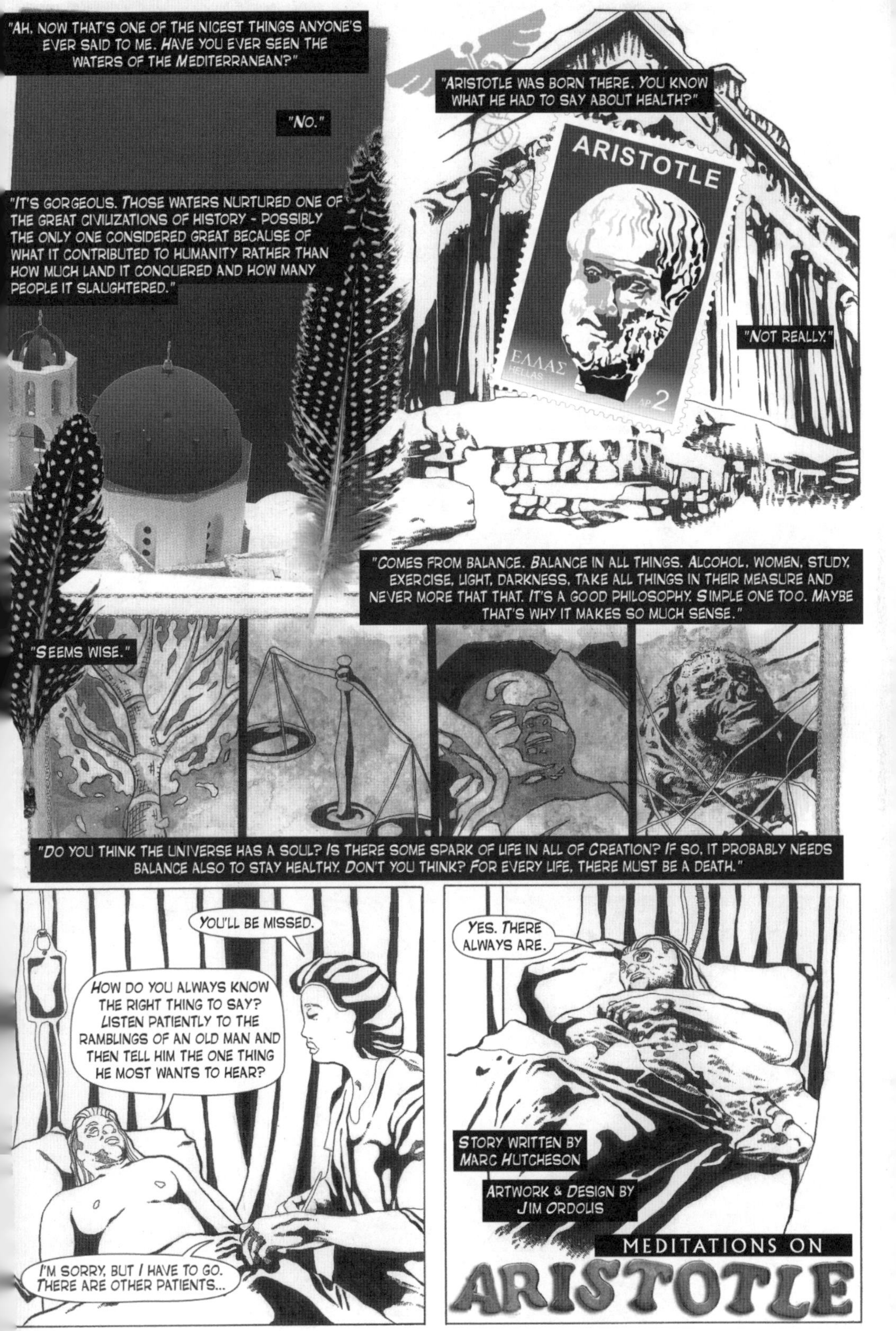
"AH, NOW THAT'S ONE OF THE NICEST THINGS ANYONE'S EVER SAID TO ME. HAVE YOU EVER SEEN THE WATERS OF THE MEDITERRANEAN?"
"NO."
"IT'S GORGEOUS. THOSE WATERS NURTURED ONE OF THE GREAT CIVILIZATIONS OF HISTORY - POSSIBLY THE ONLY ONE CONSIDERED GREAT BECAUSE OF WHAT IT CONTRIBUTED TO HUMANITY RATHER THAN HOW MUCH LAND IT CONQUERED AND HOW MANY PEOPLE IT SLAUGHTERED."
"ARISTOTLE WAS BORN THERE. YOU KNOW WHAT HE HAD TO SAY ABOUT HEALTH?"
ARISTOTLE
ΕΛΛΑΣ
HELLAS
ΔΡ 2
"NOT REALLY."
"COMES FROM BALANCE. BALANCE IN ALL THINGS. ALCOHOL, WOMEN, STUDY, EXERCISE, LIGHT, DARKNESS, TAKE ALL THINGS IN THEIR MEASURE AND NEVER MORE THAT THAT. IT'S A GOOD PHILOSOPHY. SIMPLE ONE TOO. MAYBE THAT'S WHY IT MAKES SO MUCH SENSE."
"SEEMS WISE."
"DO YOU THINK THE UNIVERSE HAS A SOUL? IS THERE SOME SPARK OF LIFE IN ALL OF CREATION? IF SO, IT PROBABLY NEEDS BALANCE ALSO TO STAY HEALTHY. DON'T YOU THINK? FOR EVERY LIFE, THERE MUST BE A DEATH."
YOU'LL BE MISSED.
HOW DO YOU ALWAYS KNOW THE RIGHT THING TO SAY? LISTEN PATIENTLY TO THE RAMBLINGS OF AN OLD MAN AND THEN TELL HIM THE ONE THING HE MOST WANTS TO HEAR?
I'M SORRY, BUT I HAVE TO GO. THERE ARE OTHER PATIENTS...
YES. THERE ALWAYS ARE.
STORY WRITTEN BY MARC HUTCHESON
ARTWORK & DESIGN BY JIM ORDOLIS
MEDITATIONS ON
ARISTOTLE

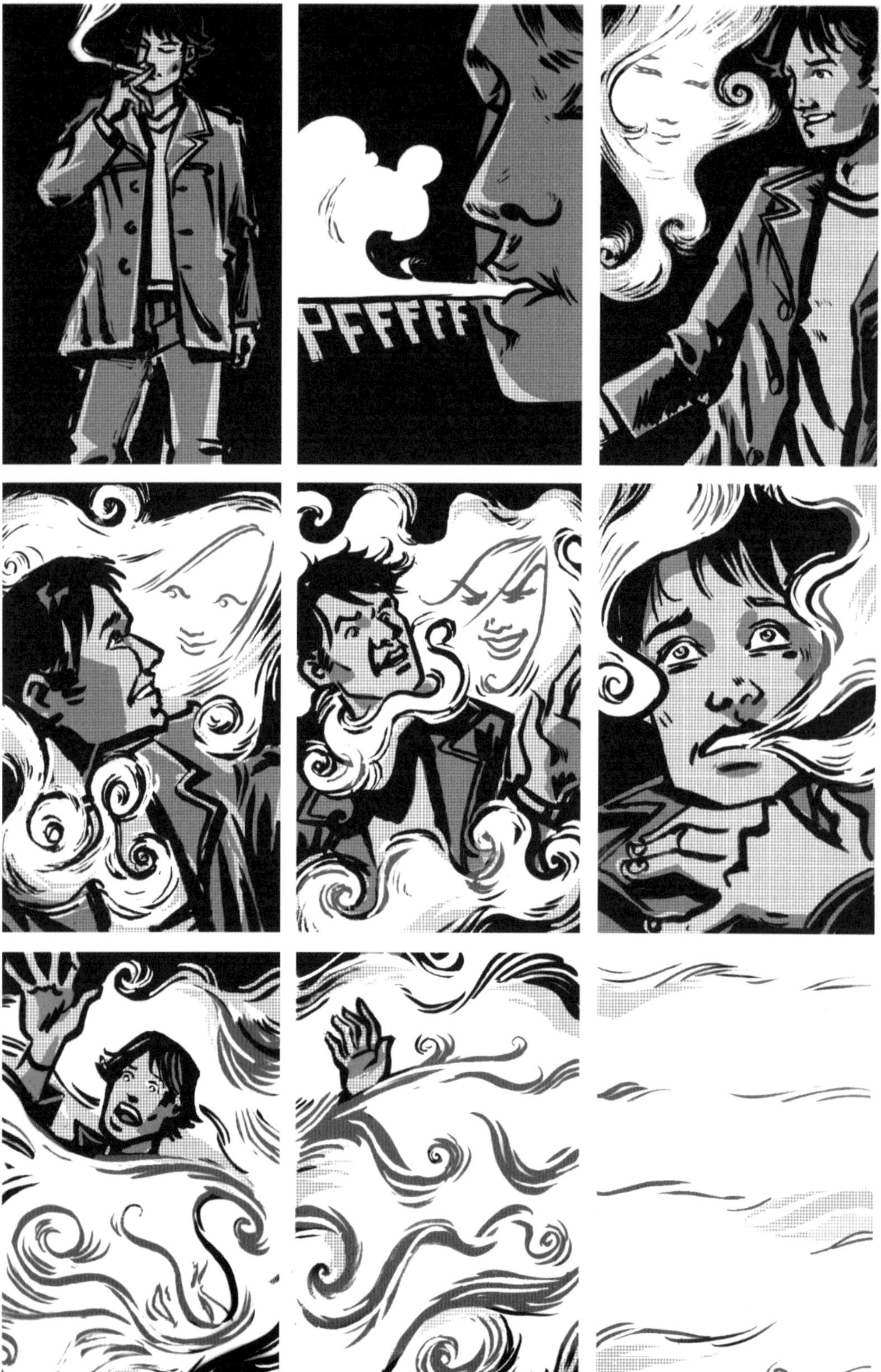
PFFFFF

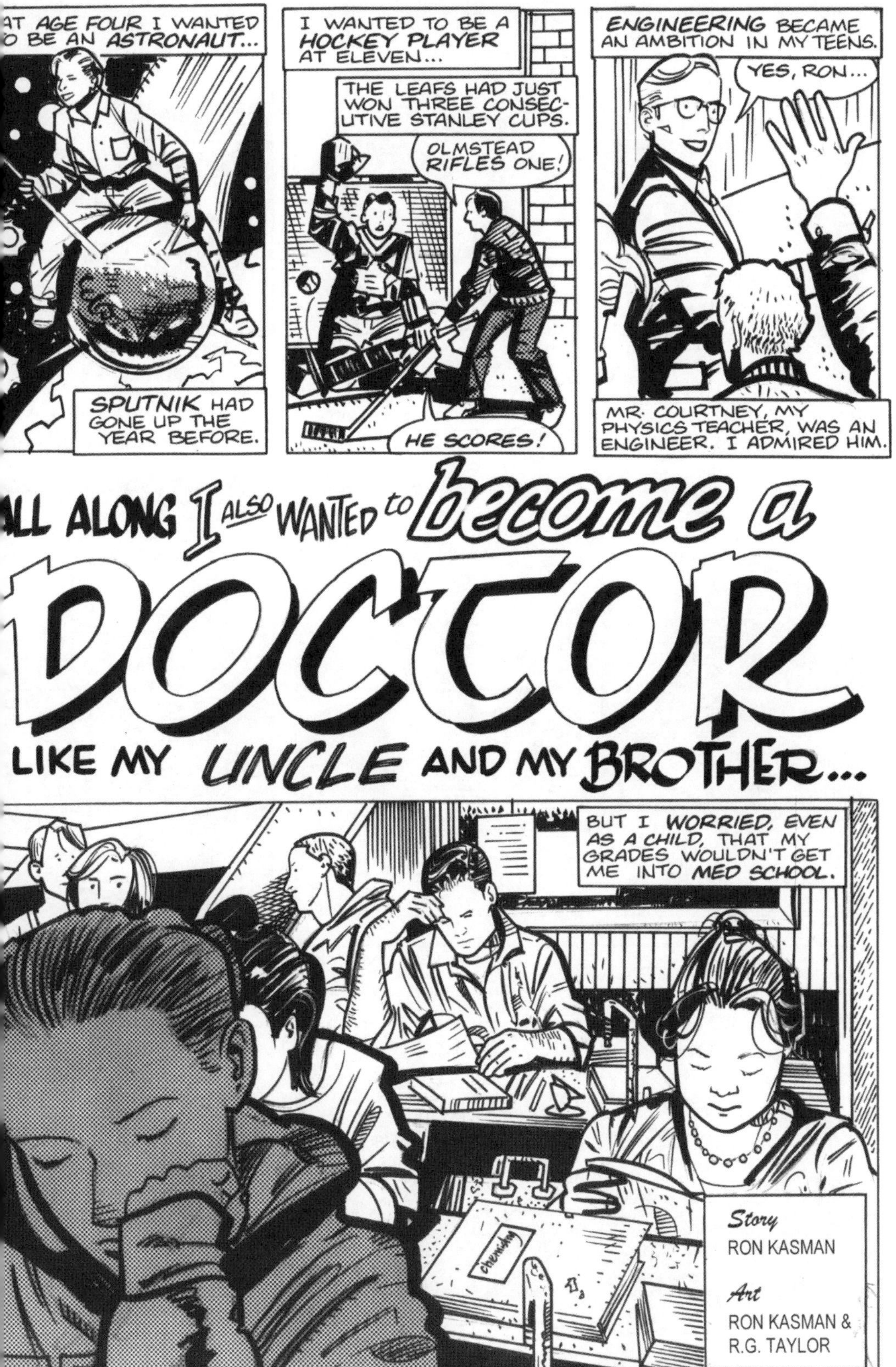
AT AGE FOUR I WANTED
O BE AN ASTRONAUT...
SPUTNIK HAD GONE UP THE YEAR BEFORE.
I WANTED TO BE A HOCKEY PLAYER AT ELEVEN...
THE LEAFS HAD JUST WON THREE CONSECUTIVE STANLEY CUPS.
OLMSTEAD RIFLES ONE!
HE SCORES!
ENGINEERING BECAME AN AMBITION IN MY TEENS.
YES, RON...
MR. COURTNEY, MY PHYSICS TEACHER, WAS AN ENGINEER. I ADMIRED HIM.
LL ALONG I ALSO WANTED to become a
DOCTOR
LIKE MY UNCLE AND MY BROTHER...
BUT I WORRIED, EVEN AS A CHILD, THAT MY GRADES WOULDN'T GET ME INTO MED SCHOOL.
chemistry
Story
RON KASMAN
Art
RON KASMAN &
R.G. TAYLOR

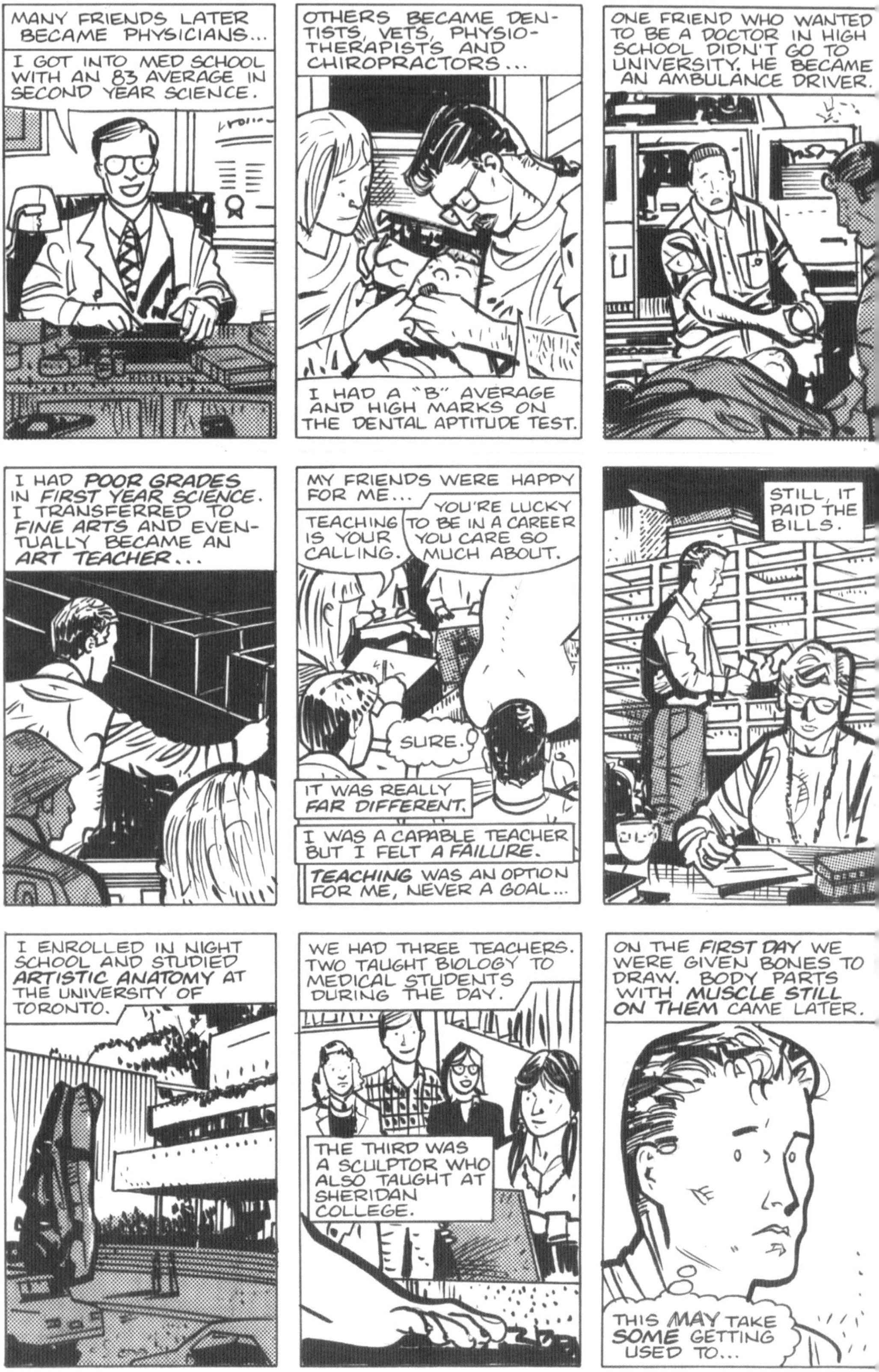
MANY FRIENDS LATER BECAME PHYSICIANS...
I GOT INTO MED SCHOOL WITH AN 83 AVERAGE IN SECOND YEAR SCIENCE.
OTHERS BECAME DENTISTS, VETS, PHYSIOTHERAPISTS AND CHIROPRACTORS...
I HAD A "B" AVERAGE AND HIGH MARKS ON THE DENTAL APTITUDE TEST.
ONE FRIEND WHO WANTED TO BE A DOCTOR IN HIGH SCHOOL DIDN'T GO TO UNIVERSITY. HE BECAME AN AMBULANCE DRIVER.
I HAD POOR GRADES IN FIRST YEAR SCIENCE. I TRANSFERRED TO FINE ARTS AND EVENTUALLY BECAME AN ART TEACHER...
MY FRIENDS WERE HAPPY FOR ME...
TEACHING IS YOUR CALLING.
YOU'RE LUCKY TO BE IN A CAREER YOU CARE SO MUCH ABOUT.
SURE.
IT WAS REALLY FAR DIFFERENT.
I WAS A CAPABLE TEACHER BUT I FELT A FAILURE.
TEACHING WAS AN OPTION FOR ME, NEVER A GOAL...
STILL, IT PAID THE BILLS.
I ENROLLED IN NIGHT SCHOOL AND STUDIED ARTISTIC ANATOMY AT THE UNIVERSITY OF TORONTO.
WE HAD THREE TEACHERS. TWO TAUGHT BIOLOGY TO MEDICAL STUDENTS DURING THE DAY.
THE THIRD WAS A SCULPTOR WHO ALSO TAUGHT AT SHERIDAN COLLEGE.
ON THE FIRST DAY WE WERE GIVEN BONES TO DRAW. BODY PARTS WITH MUSCLE STILL ON THEM CAME LATER.
THIS MAY TAKE SOME GETTING USED TO...

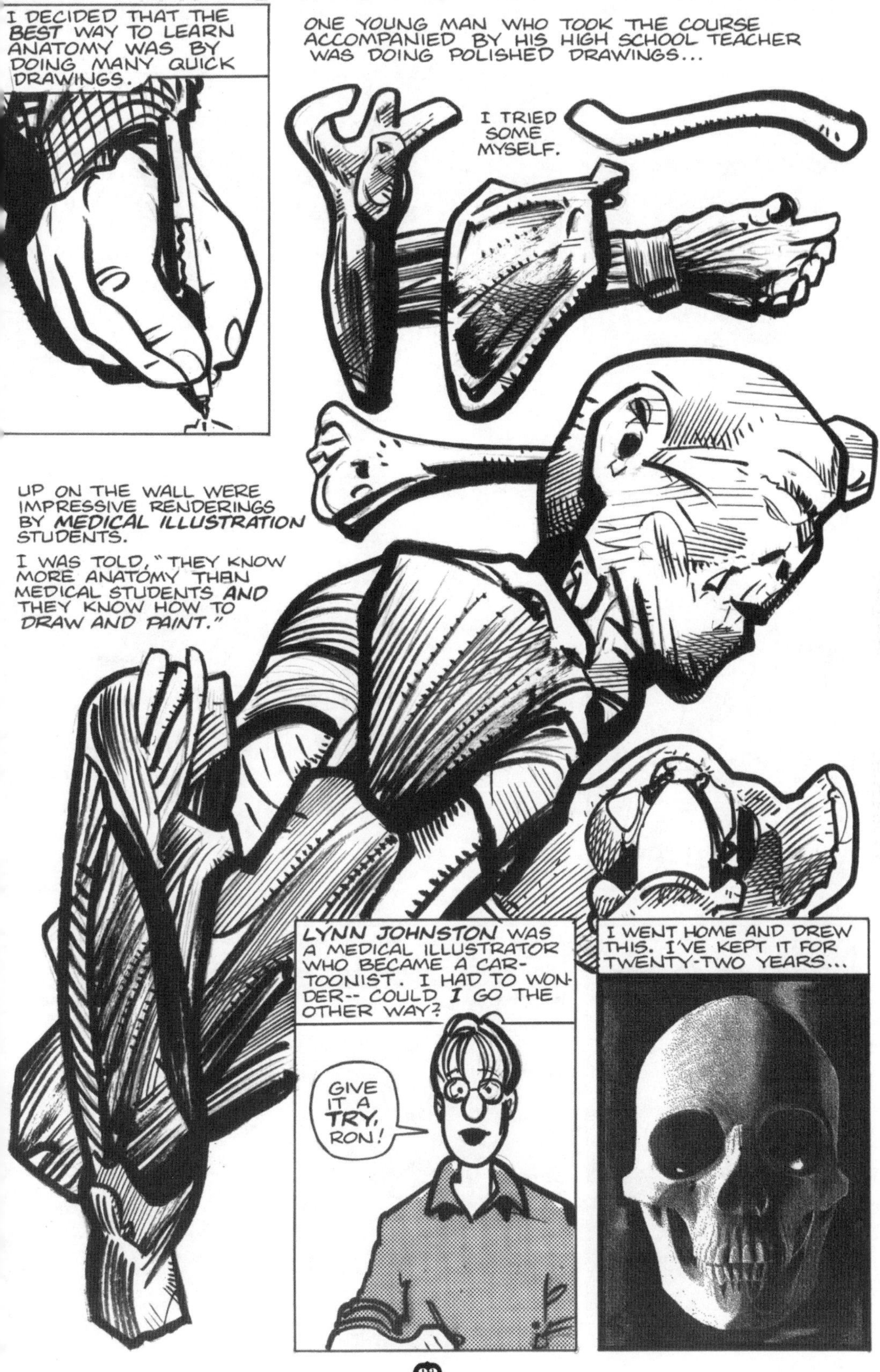
I DECIDED THAT THE BEST WAY TO LEARN ANATOMY WAS BY DOING MANY QUICK DRAWINGS.
ONE YOUNG MAN WHO TOOK THE COURSE ACCOMPANIED BY HIS HIGH SCHOOL TEACHER WAS DOING POLISHED DRAWINGS...
I TRIED SOME MYSELF.
UP ON THE WALL WERE IMPRESSIVE RENDERINGS BY MEDICAL ILLUSTRATION STUDENTS.
I WAS TOLD, "THEY KNOW MORE ANATOMY THAN MEDICAL STUDENTS AND THEY KNOW HOW TO DRAW AND PAINT."
LYNN JOHNSTON WAS A MEDICAL ILLUSTRATOR WHO BECAME A CARTOONIST. I HAD TO WONDER-- COULD I GO THE OTHER WAY?
GIVE IT A TRY, RON!
I WENT HOME AND DREW THIS. I'VE KEPT IT FOR TWENTY-TWO YEARS...

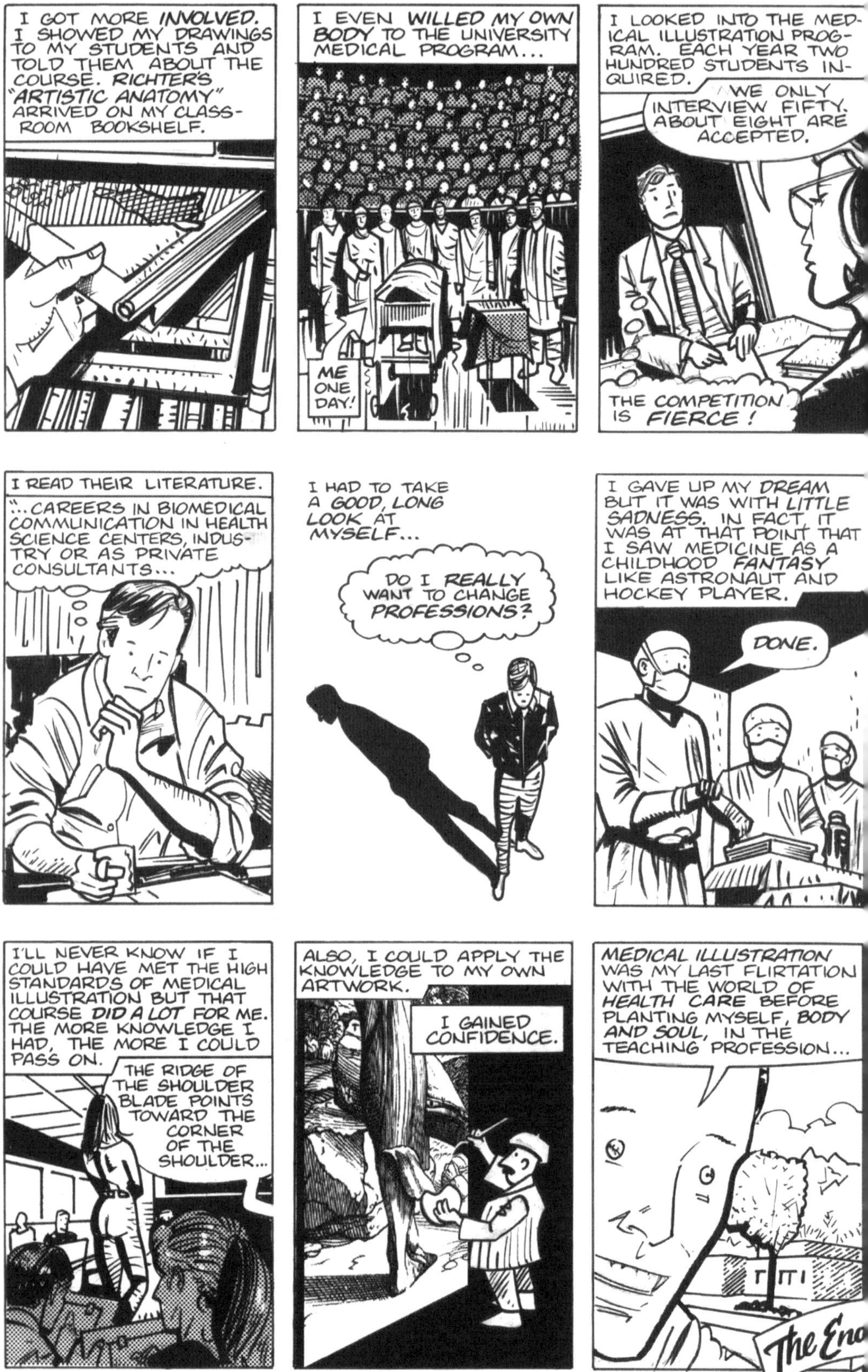

I GOT MORE INVOLVED. I SHOWED MY DRAWINGS TO MY STUDENTS AND TOLD THEM ABOUT THE COURSE. RICHTER'S "ARTISTIC ANATOMY" ARRIVED ON MY CLASSROOM BOOKSHELF.
I EVEN WILLED MY OWN BODY TO THE UNIVERSITY MEDICAL PROGRAM...
ME ONE DAY!
I LOOKED INTO THE MEDICAL ILLUSTRATION PROGRAM. EACH YEAR TWO HUNDRED STUDENTS INQUIRED.
WE ONLY INTERVIEW FIFTY. ABOUT EIGHT ARE ACCEPTED.
THE COMPETITION IS FIERCE!
I READ THEIR LITERATURE.
"...CAREERS IN BIOMEDICAL COMMUNICATION IN HEALTH SCIENCE CENTERS, INDUSTRY OR AS PRIVATE CONSULTANTS...
I HAD TO TAKE A GOOD, LONG LOOK AT MYSELF...
DO I REALLY WANT TO CHANGE PROFESSIONS?
I GAVE UP MY DREAM BUT IT WAS WITH LITTLE SADNESS. IN FACT, IT WAS AT THAT POINT THAT I SAW MEDICINE AS A CHILDHOOD FANTASY LIKE ASTRONAUT AND HOCKEY PLAYER.
DONE.
I'LL NEVER KNOW IF I COULD HAVE MET THE HIGH STANDARDS OF MEDICAL ILLUSTRATION BUT THAT COURSE DID A LOT FOR ME. THE MORE KNOWLEDGE I HAD, THE MORE I COULD PASS ON.
THE RIDGE OF THE SHOULDER BLADE POINTS TOWARD THE CORNER OF THE SHOULDER...
ALSO, I COULD APPLY THE KNOWLEDGE TO MY OWN ARTWORK.
I GAINED CONFIDENCE.
MEDICAL ILLUSTRATION WAS MY LAST FLIRTATION WITH THE WORLD OF HEALTH CARE BEFORE PLANTING MYSELF, BODY AND SOUL, IN THE TEACHING PROFESSION...

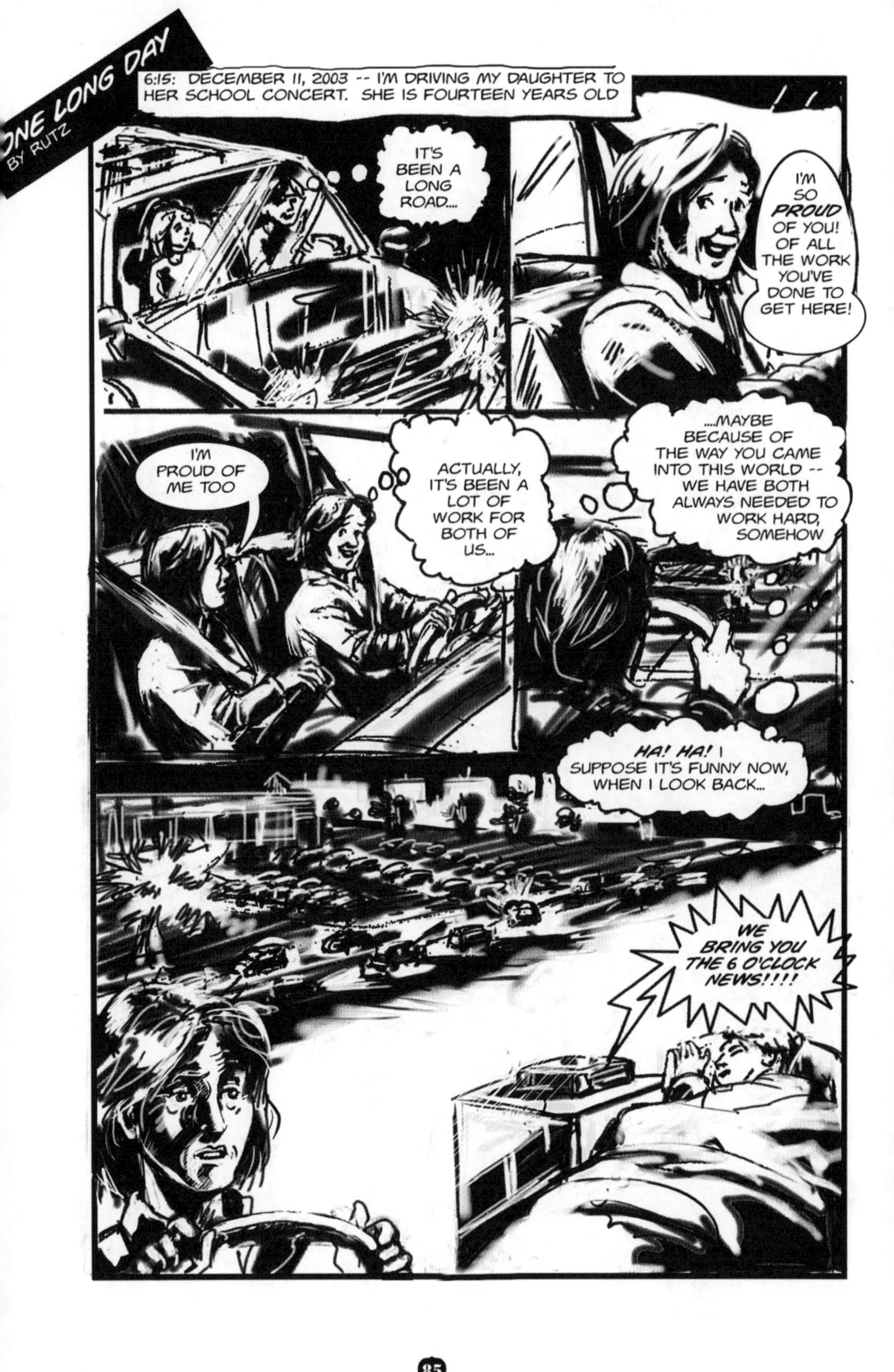
ONE LONG DAY
BY RUTZ
6:15: DECEMBER 11, 2003 -- I'M DRIVING MY DAUGHTER TO HER SCHOOL CONCERT. SHE IS FOURTEEN YEARS OLD
IT'S BEEN A LONG ROAD...
I'M SO PROUD OF YOU! OF ALL THE WORK YOU'VE DONE TO GET HERE!
I'M PROUD OF ME TOO
ACTUALLY, IT'S BEEN A LOT OF WORK FOR BOTH OF US...
...MAYBE BECAUSE OF THE WAY YOU CAME INTO THIS WORLD -- WE HAVE BOTH ALWAYS NEEDED TO WORK HARD, SOMEHOW
HA! HA! I SUPPOSE IT'S FUNNY NOW, WHEN I LOOK BACK...
WE BRING YOU THE 6 O'CLOCK NEWS!!!!

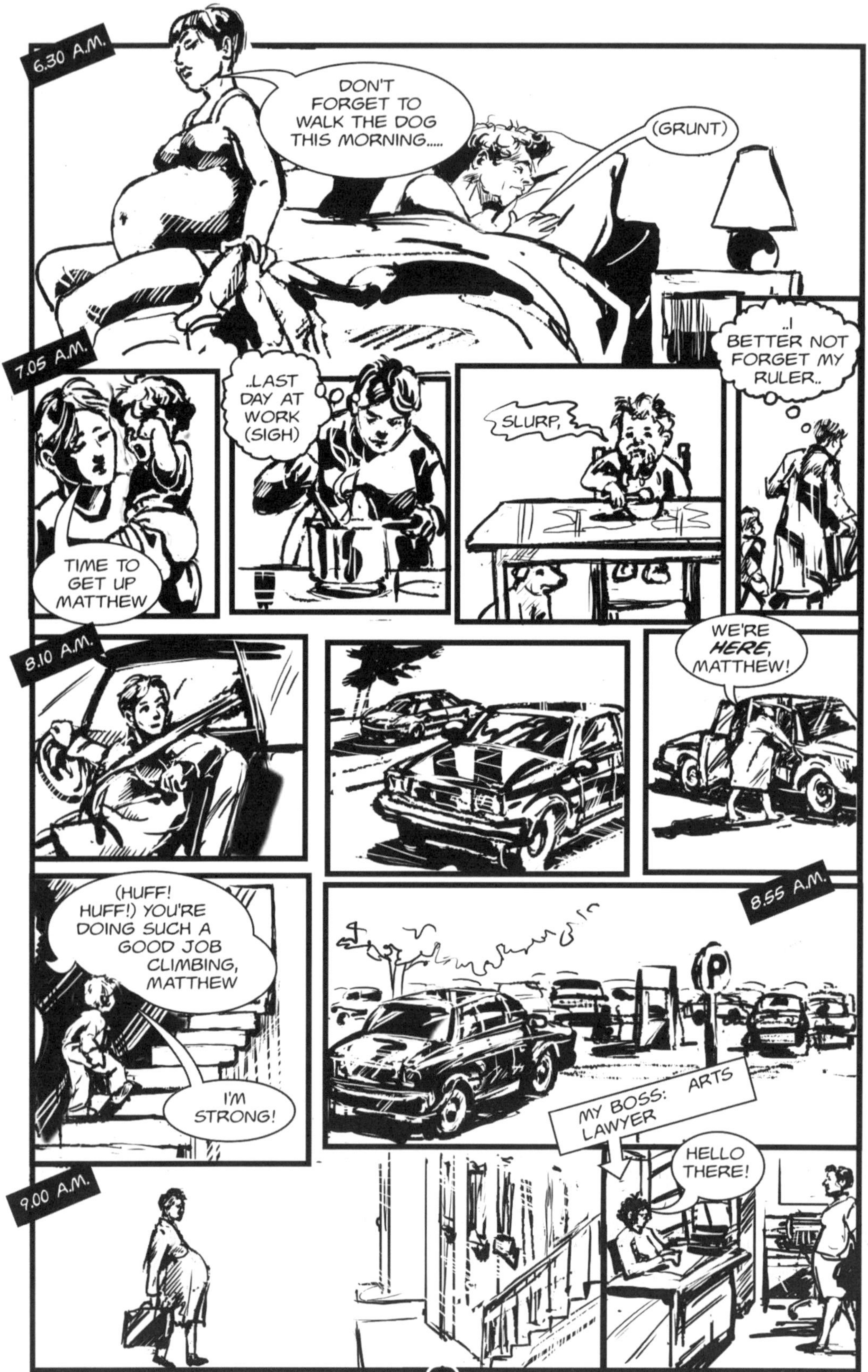
6.30 A.M.
DON'T FORGET TO WALK THE DOG THIS MORNING.....
(GRUNT)
7.05 A.M.
TIME TO GET UP MATTHEW
..LAST DAY AT WORK (SIGH)
SLURP,
..I BETTER NOT FORGET MY RULER..
8.10 A.M.
WE'RE *HERE*, MATTHEW!
(HUFF! HUFF!) YOU'RE DOING SUCH A GOOD JOB CLIMBING, MATTHEW
I'M STRONG!
8.55 A.M.
9.00 A.M.
MY BOSS: ARTS LAWYER
HELLO THERE!

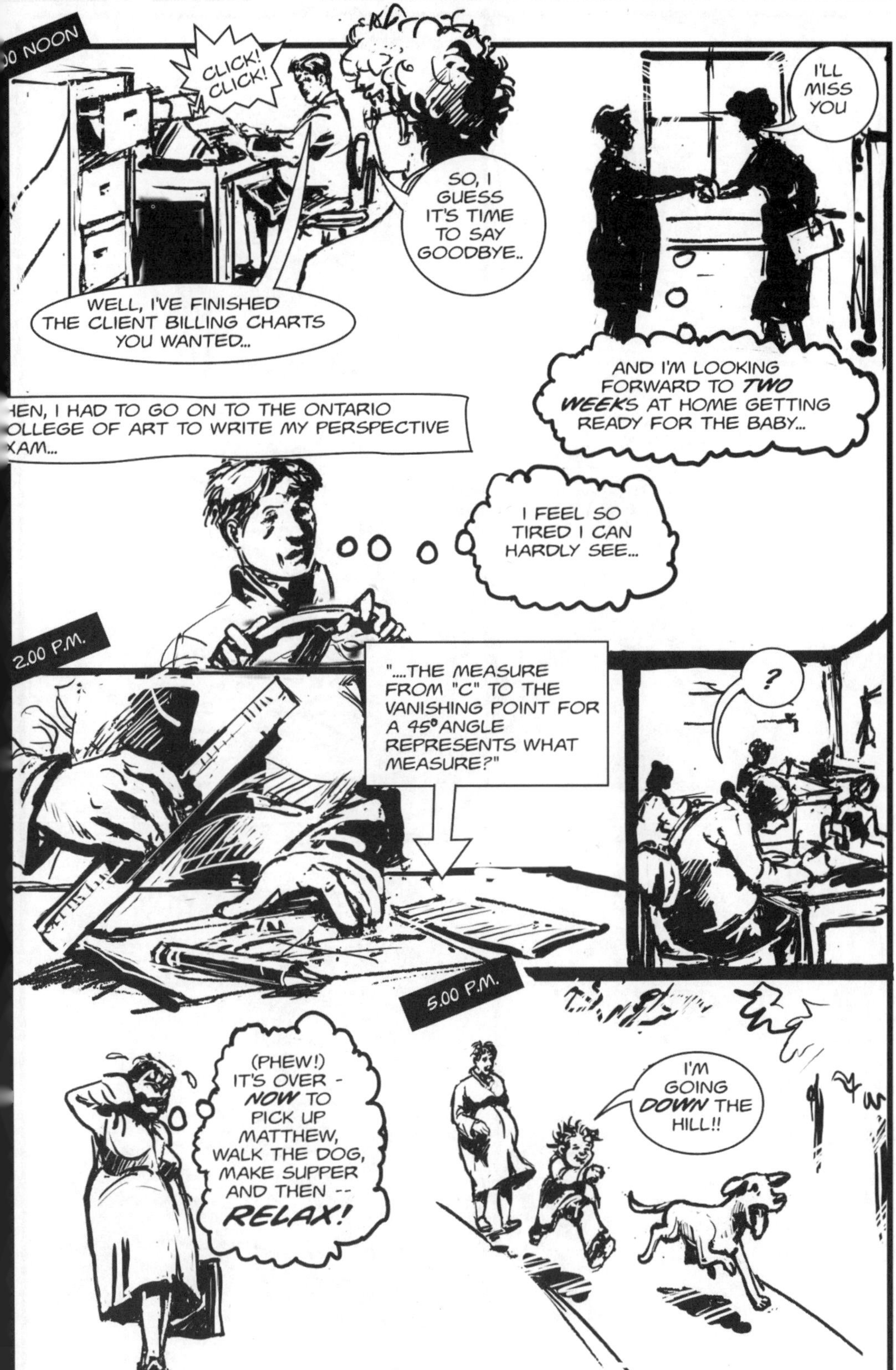

0 NOON
CLICK! CLICK!
SO, I GUESS IT'S TIME TO SAY GOODBYE..
WELL, I'VE FINISHED THE CLIENT BILLING CHARTS YOU WANTED...
I'LL MISS YOU
AND I'M LOOKING FORWARD TO TWO WEEKS AT HOME GETTING READY FOR THE BABY...
HEN, I HAD TO GO ON TO THE ONTARIO OLLEGE OF ART TO WRITE MY PERSPECTIVE XAM...
I FEEL SO TIRED I CAN HARDLY SEE...
2.00 P.M.
"....THE MEASURE FROM "C" TO THE VANISHING POINT FOR A 45° ANGLE REPRESENTS WHAT MEASURE?"
?
5.00 P.M.
(PHEW!) IT'S OVER - NOW TO PICK UP MATTHEW, WALK THE DOG, MAKE SUPPER AND THEN -- RELAX!
I'M GOING DOWN THE HILL!!

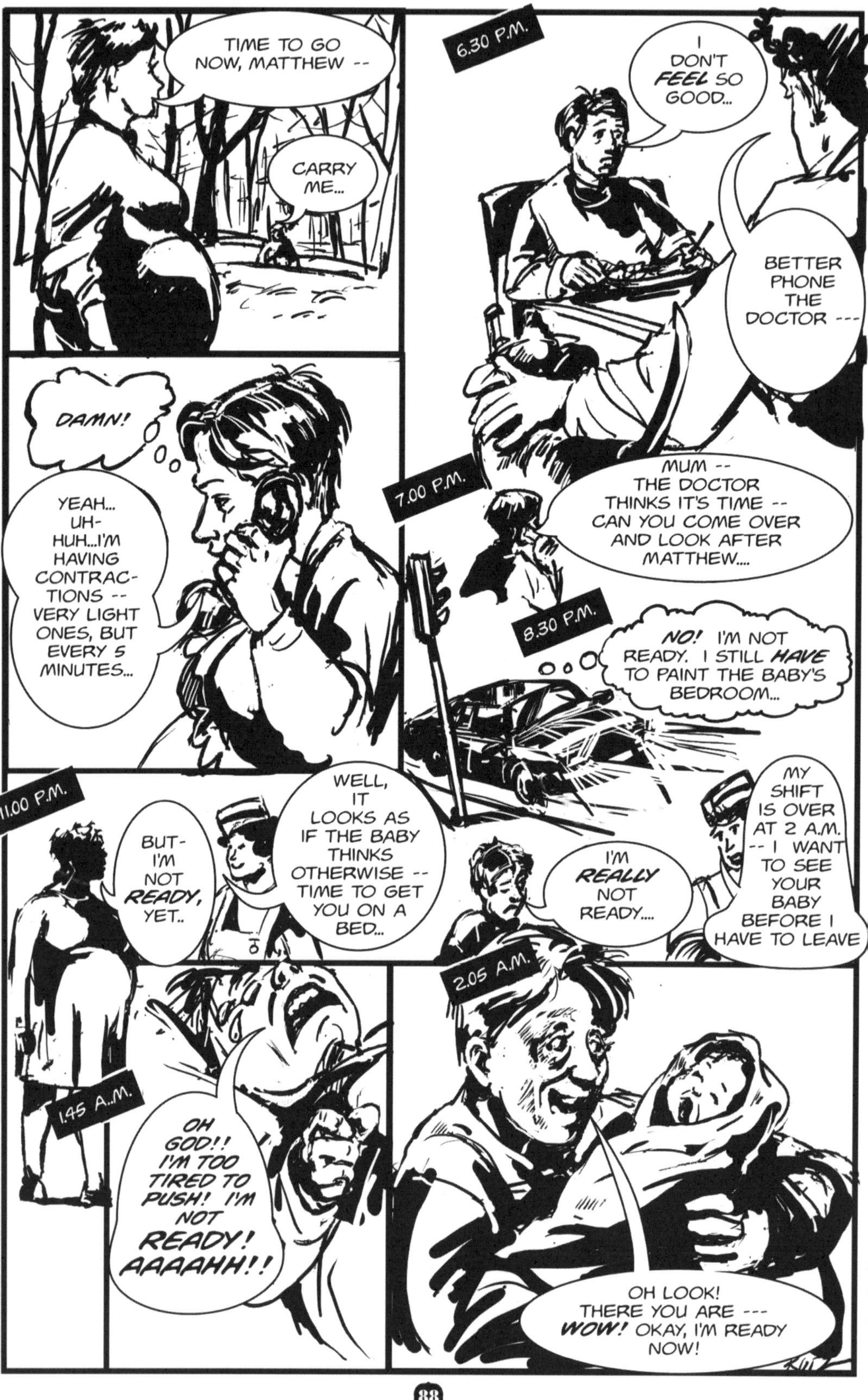
TIME TO GO NOW, MATTHEW --
CARRY ME...
6.30 P.M.
I DON'T FEEL SO GOOD...
BETTER PHONE THE DOCTOR ---
DAMN!
YEAH... UH-HUH...I'M HAVING CONTRAC-TIONS -- VERY LIGHT ONES, BUT EVERY 5 MINUTES...
7.00 P.M.
MUM -- THE DOCTOR THINKS IT'S TIME -- CAN YOU COME OVER AND LOOK AFTER MATTHEW....
8.30 P.M.
NO! I'M NOT READY. I STILL HAVE TO PAINT THE BABY'S BEDROOM...
11.00 P.M.
BUT- I'M NOT READY, YET..
WELL, IT LOOKS AS IF THE BABY THINKS OTHERWISE -- TIME TO GET YOU ON A BED...
I'M REALLY NOT READY....
MY SHIFT IS OVER AT 2 A.M. -- I WANT TO SEE YOUR BABY BEFORE I HAVE TO LEAVE
1.45 A.M.
OH GOD!! I'M TOO TIRED TO PUSH! I'M NOT READY! AAAAHH!!
2.05 A.M.
OH LOOK! THERE YOU ARE --- WOW! OKAY, I'M READY NOW!

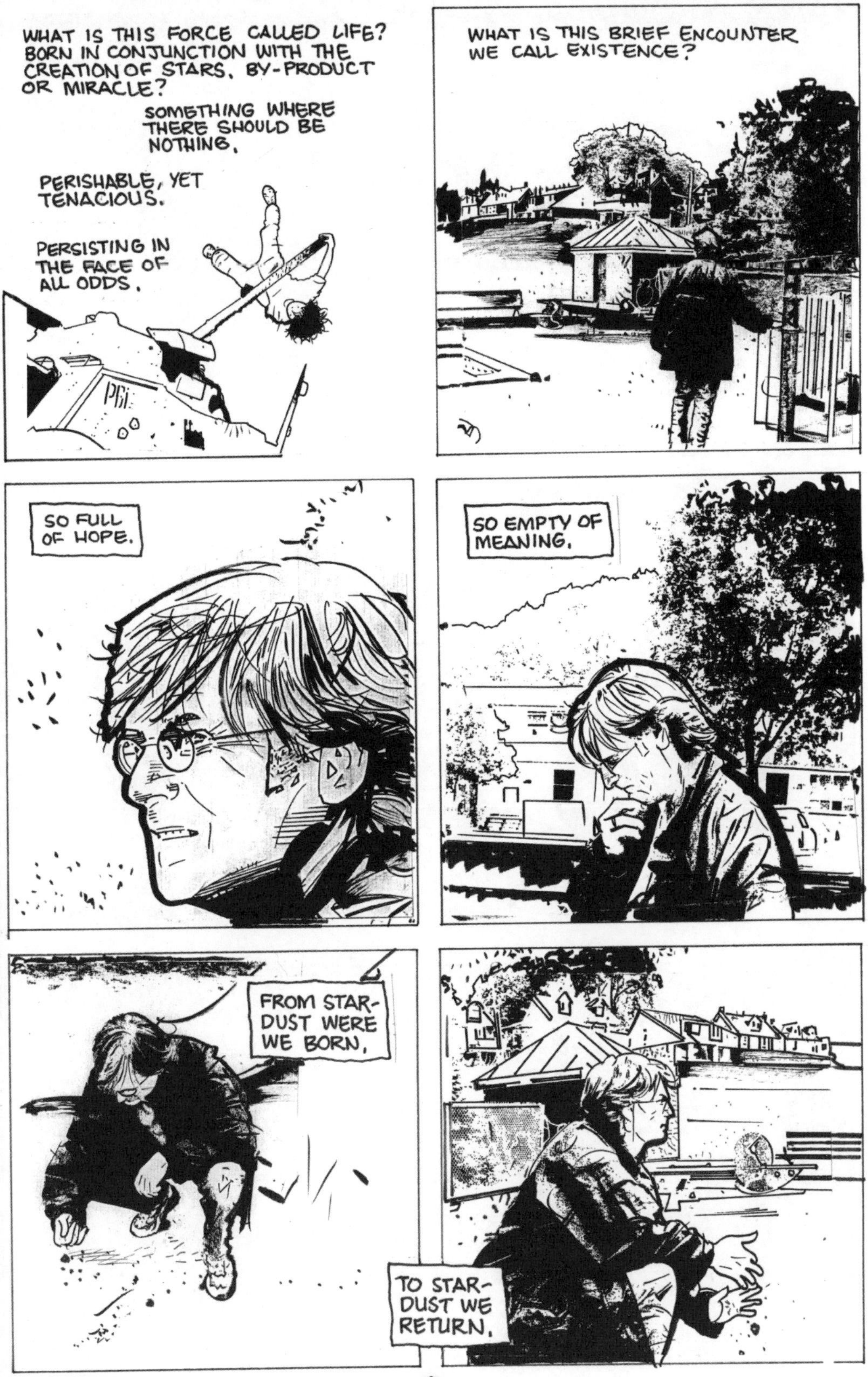
WHAT IS THIS FORCE CALLED LIFE? BORN IN CONJUNCTION WITH THE CREATION OF STARS. BY-PRODUCT OR MIRACLE?
SOMETHING WHERE THERE SHOULD BE NOTHING.
PERISHABLE, YET TENACIOUS.
PERSISTING IN THE FACE OF ALL ODDS.
WHAT IS THIS BRIEF ENCOUNTER WE CALL EXISTENCE?
SO FULL OF HOPE.
SO EMPTY OF MEANING.
FROM STAR-DUST WERE WE BORN.
TO STAR-DUST WE RETURN.

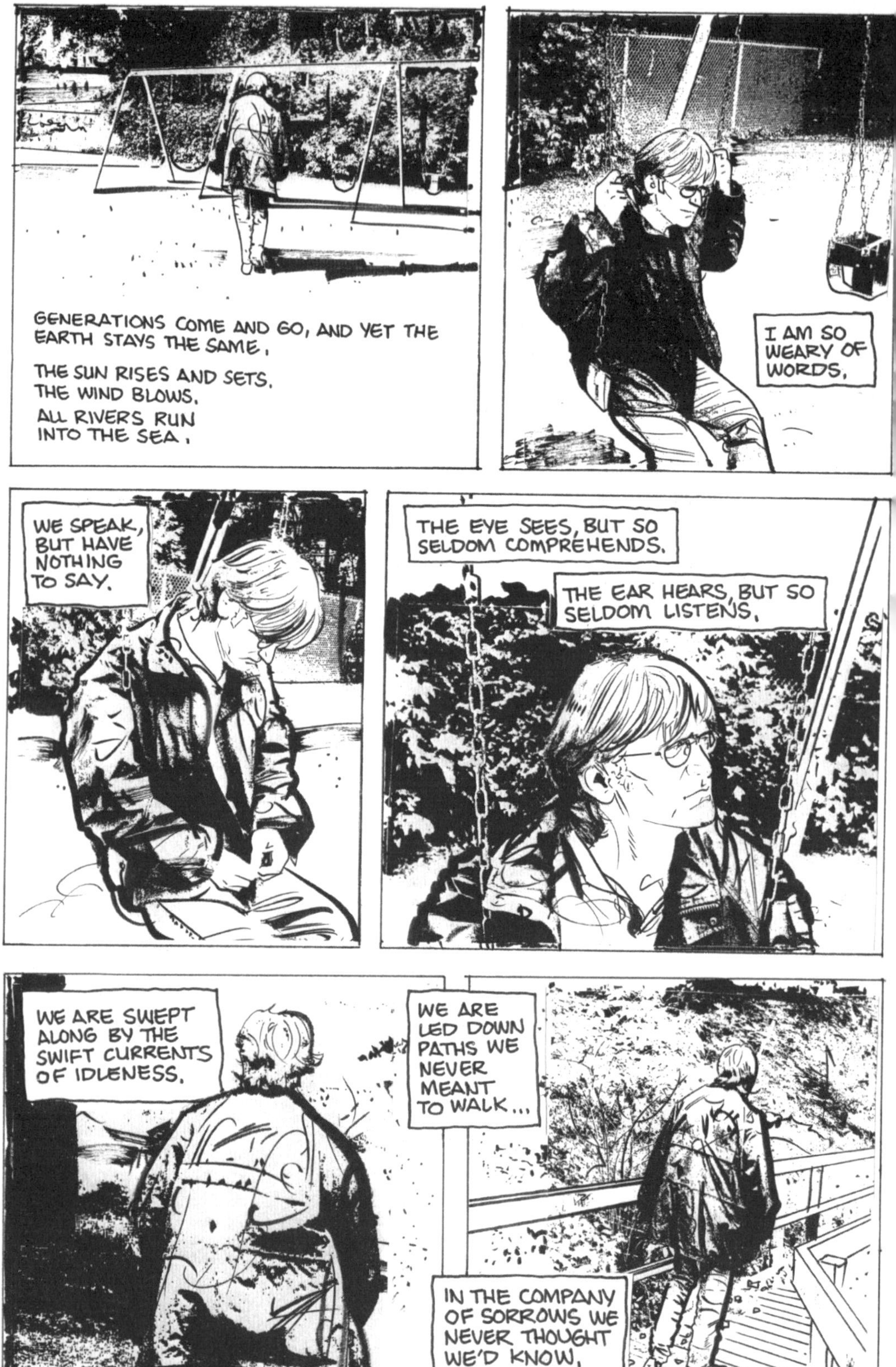
GENERATIONS COME AND GO, AND YET THE EARTH STAYS THE SAME.
THE SUN RISES AND SETS.
THE WIND BLOWS.
ALL RIVERS RUN INTO THE SEA.
I AM SO WEARY OF WORDS.
WE SPEAK, BUT HAVE NOTHING TO SAY.
THE EYE SEES, BUT SO SELDOM COMPREHENDS.
THE EAR HEARS, BUT SO SELDOM LISTENS.
WE ARE SWEPT ALONG BY THE SWIFT CURRENTS OF IDLENESS.
WE ARE LED DOWN PATHS WE NEVER MEANT TO WALK...
IN THE COMPANY OF SORROWS WE NEVER THOUGHT WE'D KNOW.

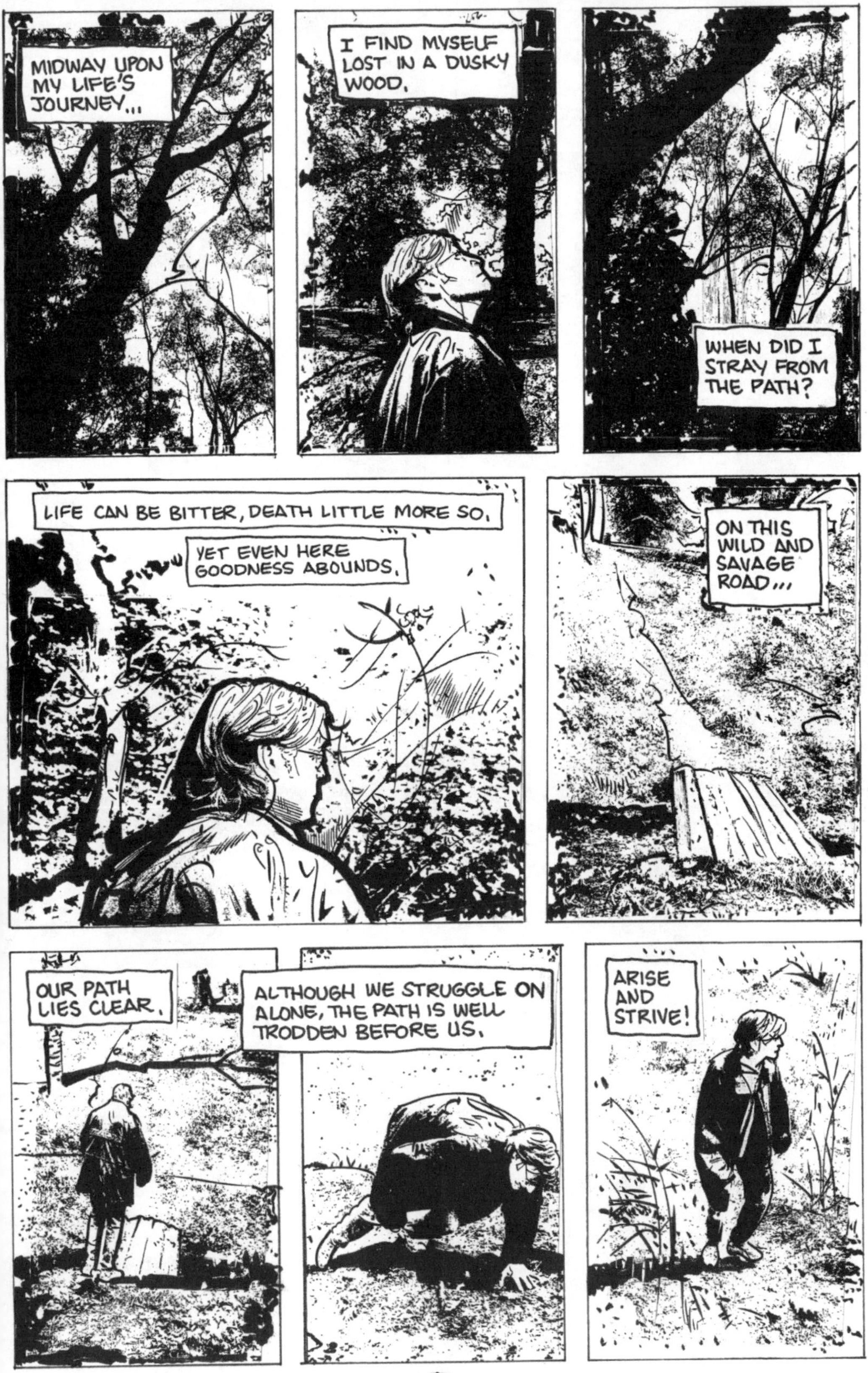
MIDWAY UPON MY LIFE'S JOURNEY...
I FIND MYSELF LOST IN A DUSKY WOOD.
WHEN DID I STRAY FROM THE PATH?
LIFE CAN BE BITTER, DEATH LITTLE MORE SO.
YET EVEN HERE GOODNESS ABOUNDS.
ON THIS WILD AND SAVAGE ROAD...
OUR PATH LIES CLEAR.
ALTHOUGH WE STRUGGLE ON ALONE, THE PATH IS WELL TRODDEN BEFORE US.
ARISE AND STRIVE!

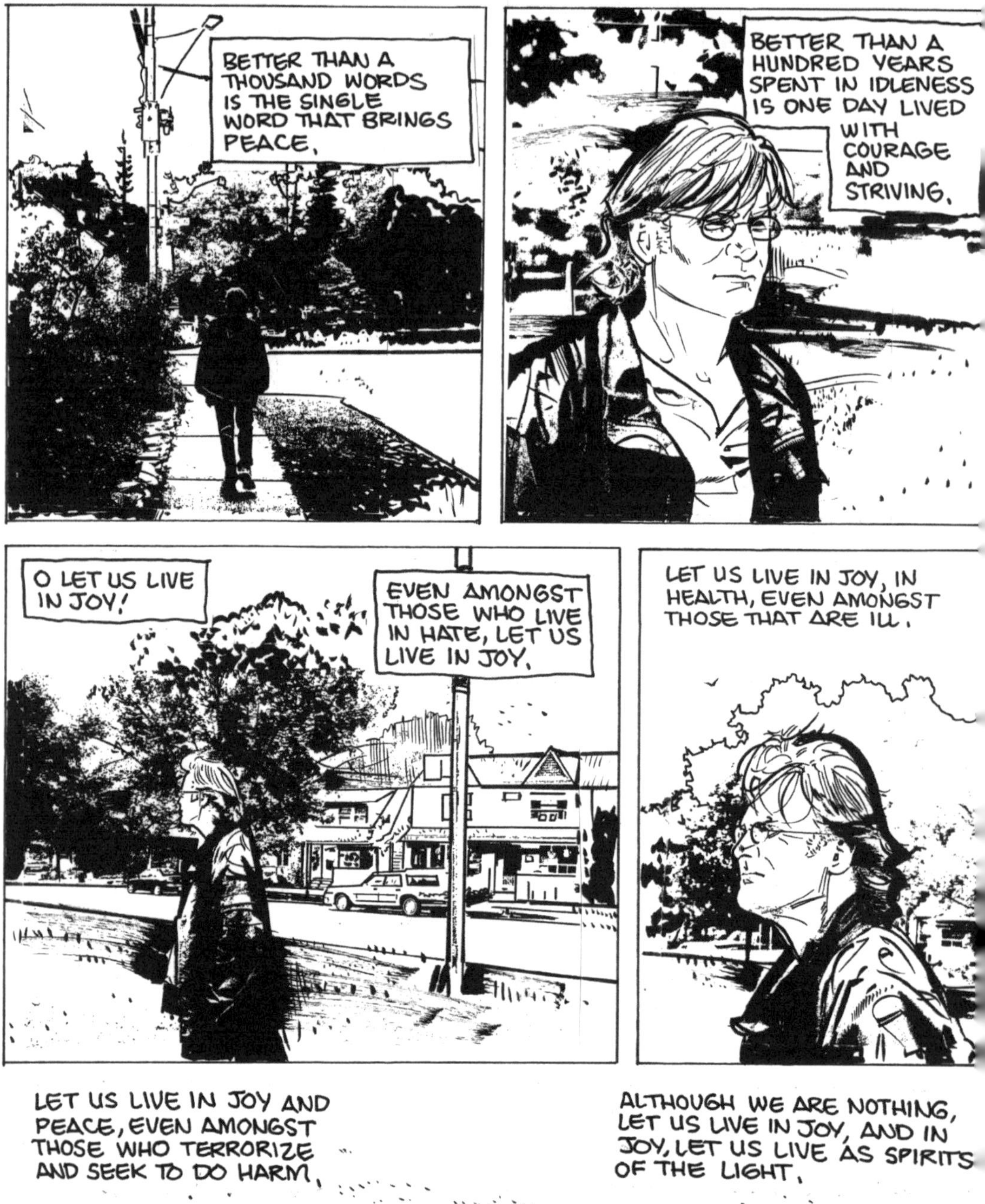

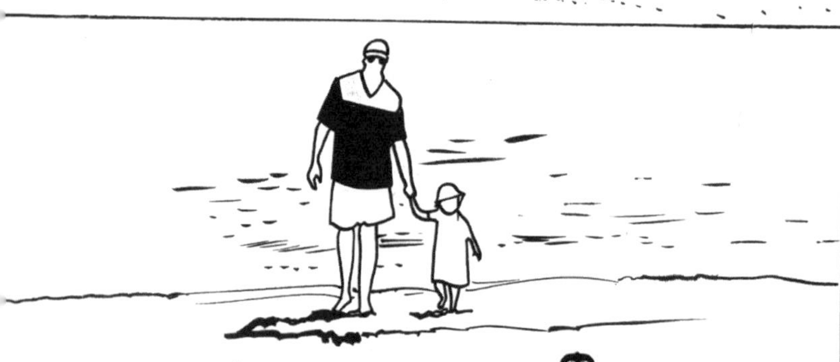

"VANITIES"

STORY, SCRIPT & LETTERING BY ROB WALTON

STORY & ART BY R.G. TAYLOR

TEXT INSPIRED BY THE DHAMMAPADA

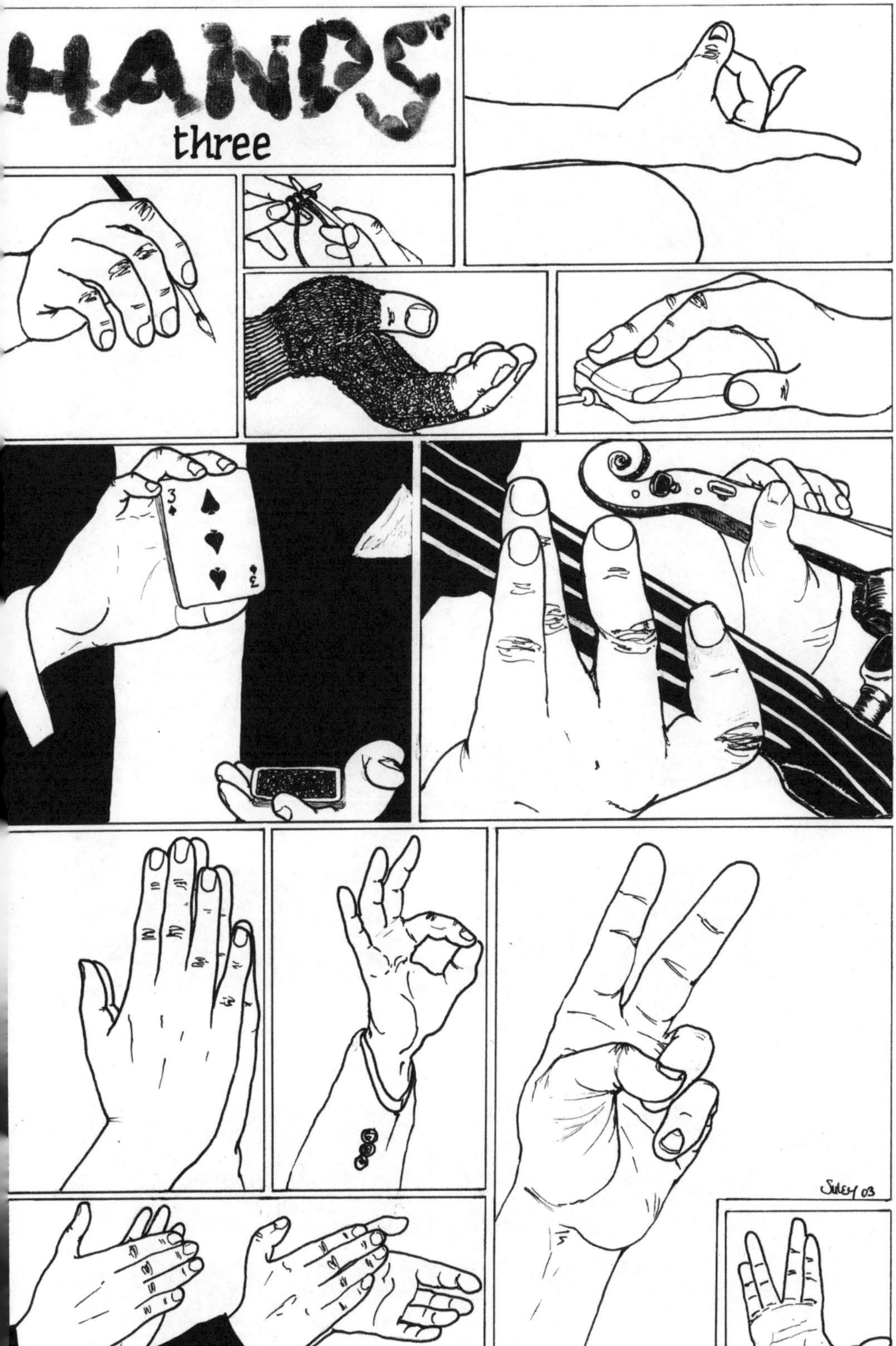
HANDS
three
Sulesy 03

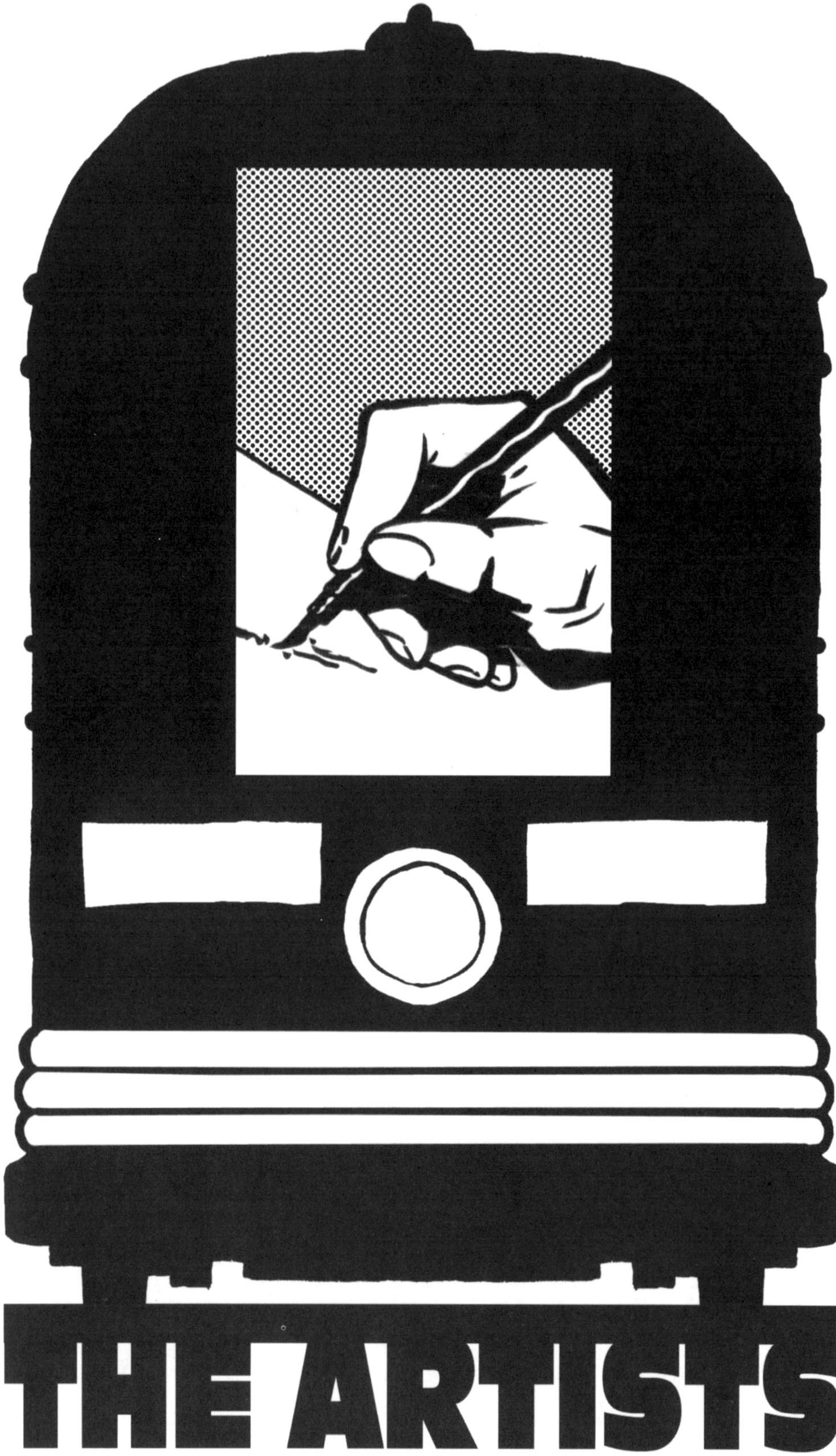

THE ARTISTS

Jason Armstrong - pgs. 68 - 71
Jason Armstrong ain't no eye-candy comic book nerd. After a gruelling 6 years workin' for Marvel, DC, Dark Horse and the like, he's currently doing life without parole at a television animation studio in downtown Toronto. He says he likes his comics pretty much like everything else; "straight up ina dirty glass." Ferro City is his latest atrocity. "I ain't sorry about nothin' I done" he says, "and I'd do it all over agin!"

Mark Askwith - pgs. 6 - 13
Mark Askwith is a comic book writer whose comics include Silencers and The Prisoner. He is also a producer for the Canadian Science Fiction Channel- SPACE: The Imagination Station.

Fred Bernard - pgs. 42 - 48
Fred was born in 1969 in Burgundy, France. After completing his university studies in sciences, he decided to try his hand at fine art. At art school he blossomed and his attention turned to honing his artistic talents. He became an author and illustrator of children's books and found a great collaboration partnership with his schoolmate, François Roca. Among his 20 plus titles, a number of them have won awards, including "Jésus Betz", which has been produced as a play by an international touring company from Chile. Fred lives in Burgundy and recently published his first adult bande dessinée, "La Tendresse des Crocodiles".

Claudia Bernhardt - pg - 60 top
Born in Lippstadt, Germany Claudia has always shown a love and interest in art and all things creative. During 1996-2000 she studied illustration and design at the University of Applied Sciences in Bielefeld, Germany; at Academie Minerva in Groningen, Netherlands and at the University of Applied Sciences in Hamburg, Germany. She has worked as a designer, an illustrator, a cartoonist, as well as working as a freelancer designer for magazines, newspapers, and corporate clients. Claudia has also created a limited illustration magazine called “Mischer”, since 1997. More about her, and her art can be seen on her web site: www.istprodukt.de.

Ron Boyd - pgs. 38 - 41, front cover
Ron Boyd has worked for Marvel, DC, and Dark Horse comics, and is an accomplished commercial illustrator. He can be found on the web at www.ronboyd.com.

Chester Brown - pgs. - 14 - 16
Chester Brown is a Canadian cartoonist living in Toronto. His graphic novels include 'Yummy Fur', 'Ed the Happy Clown', I Never Liked You', and his latest graphic novel is a biography of Louis Riel.

Dominic Bugatto - pgs. 17, 74 - 75
Dominic Bugatto was born in Bradford, West Yorkshire, England. While he works primarily as an illustrator, Dominic has also included stints as a designer and concept artist for both film and television. His clients have included The L.A. Times, Washington Post,, Spin, Details and FHM. Visit www.dominicbugatto.com for more of Dominic's work.

David Cullen - pgs. 52 - 56
David Cullen was born in Halifax, Nova Scotia. After an 8-year stint in Texas and Maine, he returned to Halifax to attend the Nova Scotia College of Art and Design. He's worked as a freelance artist for 14 years, primarily doing storyboards and comics. Some of his earliest work was for Marvel Comics and Salter Street Films' sci-fi cult-hit, "Lexx". He's since worked for numerous film production companies and advertising agencies, but remains most proud of his comic book work. His most recent comics story(prior to this one) was in the anthology one-shot, "Frecklebean Comics and Stories".

Willow Dawson - pgs. 58 - 59
Willow spent many years in and out of the hospital as a young girl in Vancouver, BC. She missed many school days but life was not sad for little Willow... she had all the backyard bugs and her imaginary friend the "Gargoyle" for company. She had her wonderful dad who taught her how to draw and to be creative. She had the beach and it's endless empty surf, the woods and the mountains of BC. Willow is very glad she grew up with asthma, because without it, she wouldn't be half the person she is today. Willow can be contacted at whoisjezebelle@hotmail.com. See her art: www.shebytches.com/willowsartpg1.html

Suley Fattah - pgs. 37, 61, 93
Suley Fattah is the dreamer who conjured this project, Drawing The Line. His passion for comics and bande dessinée spawned the idea of this fundraising effort. His life is equally creative: he works predominantly in the magic field assisting various magicians, on stage and off. Recently he has illustrated over 220 images for a monthly magic periodical and over 150 images for a magic book.

Marcel Guldemond - pgs. 18 - 21
Marcel currently lives in Eastern Ontario. He really likes drawing comics, but he doesn't like commuting in the morning very much at all. He posts online comics at the fantastic serializer website: http://www.serializer.net. Information about his corporeal comics and art can be found at http://aporia.brainmade.com

Janet Hetherington - pgs. 76 - 77
Janet Hetherington is a writer/cartoonist with a degree in Journalism from Carleton University in Ottawa, Canada. Janet is the creator, writer and artist of Eternal Romance, a supernatural romance comic book, and she is currently writing the adventures of Elvira, Mistress of the Dark for Claypool Comics. In 1999, Janet received Canada's Aurora Award for excellence in science fiction and fantasy. Janet lives in Ottawa where she shares a studio with artist Ronn Sutton.

Marc Hutcheson - pgs. 78 - 79
Marc Hutcheson currently resides in Marina del Rey, California. He is collaborating with artist Jim Ordolis on an epic graphic novel. This tale centers on the mystic quest of a lone artist to bridge the gap between imagination and reality, and to save all of mankind from the endless trap of the human condition.

Stuart Immonen & Kathryn Kuder - pgs. 34 - 36
Stuart and Kathryn have been making comics together for a long time and have been friends for even longer than that. They live in Obscurity, Ontario with their two and four-footed family and invite you to visit them at www.immonen.ca

Ron Kasman - pgs. 81 - 84
Ron Kasman is an art teacher in Oakville, Ontario who has also worked for dozens of comic book publishing companies in the United States and Canada including Image, D.C. and Eclipse. He is one of the few artists to draw two of the comic book characters appearing on Canadian postage stamps (inks and letters on the first drawings of Fleur de Lys and pencils and letters on the Captain Canuck comic strip).

Neil Kleid - pgs. 62 - 63
Neil Kleid creates minicomics and stories when no one thinks he's awake. He's's illustrated for magazines like BIG NEWS and KITCHEN SINK while creating comics for anthologies including Alternative Comics' 9-11: EMERGENCY RELIEF, Modern Tales: Longplay,+ HOUSE OF TWELVE, MAULED! and TRUE PORN. Recently, Neil won a Xeric Grant to publish NINET CANDLES, a 48 page improvisational graphic novel about the life of a cartoonist, one panel per year. Between working on a graphic novel about Murder Inc. with artist Jake Allen for NBM Publishing, and his first play, AMERICAN CAESAR, Neil harbors notions of writing comic books full time. Weep for him.

Gisèle Laval - pg 60 bottom

Gisele Laval was born in France in 1971. She studied graphic arts and drawing for five years, at La Martinière-Terreaux and Ecole Emile Cohl (both in Lyon). In 1994 Gisele became a commercial graphic artist and painter producing signs, informational panels and billboards. Today, she designs and illustrates images of animals, flora and fauna on permanent informational panels for national parks, heritage and historical sites. She has also illustrated " Le Piqueur des Bottières" by Pierre Lieuze.

Steve LeBlanc - pgs. 50 - 51

STEVE LeBLANC is the Toronto graphic artist / illustrator of James Waley's Caliber Comics' mini-series, "Ali-Baba: Scourge of the Desert" and Dave (Wordsmith) Darrigo's crime series "Tony Bravado: Trouble-Shooter". Having explored the world of gallery artwork recently with showings of his paintings Steve is once again producing comic art on "ABOVE & BEYOND..." after reuniting with his former ALI-BABA collaborator. While not abandoning his painterly pursuits, Steve's love of the comic medium has never waned and he is currently developing a creator-owned detective series, HOGTOWN --- watch for it! (sleblanc@trader.ca)

Andy Lee - pg. 31

Andy Lee is a Modern Zen artist from Hong Kong. Zen Art originated in China (known first as Chan Buddhist art). The literati in the 13th Century Chan Dynasty were restricted to certain fine-line styles by the Emperor. The Buddhist monks revolted and painted in a loose cerebral fashion. This came to be known as Zen art. It is a process of splashing sumi ink on the page and creating images out of chaos for the purpose of self enlightenment and discovery. Andy's work is shown in many galleries worldwide. You can find his published work in Dragonball Z, Ultimate Marvel Team Ups (Spiderman vs. Master of Kung Fu), Strangers in Paradise, Kabuki, Sam and Twitch, Kindred of the East, The Crow and Anime Insider. His website is www.findandy.com.

Nick Marinkovich - pgs. 22 - 26

A graduate of University of Western Ontario, with a BSc in Genetics, Nick has since worked in Toronto as an illustrator and media designer. In 2002 he co-illustrated "The Reverie" by Daniel Fischer, with Nick Postic. Recent appearances include his co-illustration work in the graphic novel adaptation of Sony film "Underworld", for IDW Publishing, with regular partner, Nick Postic. Also, he was featured in the short story "Leviathan", published in Digital Webbing Presents (also with Postic). Currently Nick is working on Underworld miniseries for IDW, with the first issue to be released in March 2004.

Moebius - pg. 57, back cover

Jean 'Moebius' Giraud is one of the most respected and influential cartoonists in the world. He was born in Paris in 1938. In 1956, before he was 18, he drew his own comic strip, Frank et Jeremie, and early in 1961, he collaborated with Joseph Gillian on Jerry Spring, a western. This led directly to the popular western strip Blueberry, co- created and written by Jean-Michel Charlier. In 1975, as one of the founding members of Les Humanoides Associes, he helped create Metal Hurlant, a groundbreaking science fiction comic book magazine. It was repackaged in English as Heavy Metal. In the mid-eighties most of his work was re-printed by Epic comics, an imprint of Marvel Comics. Moebius has also worked on influential movies- he designed costumes for Ridley Scott's Alien and helped storyboard and design Bladerunner, *Tron* , James Cameron's *Abyss* and Luc Besson's *The Fifth Element*. Moebius is currently working on an animated movie called *Through the Moebius Strip*.

Dean Motter - pgs. 27 - 30

Triple-threat creator (writer, designer, illustrator) DEAN MOTTER is perhaps best known as the creator of the '80's comic book sensation MISTER X (the archival collection due to be published by Simon & Schuster later this year.) In 1988 he illustrated and co-wrote DC's THE PRISONER. His two highly lauded Vertigo mini-series TERMINAL CITY and TERMINAL CITY: AERIAL GRAFFITI were nominated for a number of Eisner and Kurtzman Awards in 1997 and 1998. Most recently Dean created the award-winning graphic novel BATMAN: NINE LIVES (with Michael Lark) as well as writing and illustrating the acclaimed Image Comics mini-series, ELECTROPOLIS.

Jim Ordolis - pgs. 78 - 79

Jim has been an illustrator & cartoonist since he convinced his father to spend 20 cents on Avengers #98 in 1972. In the last 10 years he's worked primarily in Graphic Arts and Web Design. Getting back to his roots, he recently contributed to Clipheart Press, Grey Anthology, Fleshrot: Tales From the Dead 2 as well as performing work for Hi Fi Color Design. He is currently working on a dark fantasy series with writer Marc Hutcheson.

Stan Sakai - pgs. 64 - 67

Stan Sakai's Usagi Yojimbo first saw print in 1984. Since then, the samurai rabbit has appeared on television as a guest of the Teenage Mutant Ninja Turtles, as toys, clothing, calendars, and a series of trade paperback collections. Among Stan's awards are a Parents Choice Award, an Inkpot, multiple Eisners, an American Library Association Award, and a National Cartoonist Society Comic Book Division Award.

Ben Shannon - pg. 80

Ben Shannon approaches his illustrations like a trendy director approaches films. Hip characters interact in cool urban settings that are always perfectly lit and creatively composed. His dynamic yet naturalistic line of work and sophisticated colour combinations create illustration with a fresh modern edge. Ben's work has spanned the fields of advertising, fashion, beauty, music, magazines, publishing, newspapers, character development and animation.

Dave Sim - pgs. 14 - 16

Dave Sim is a Canadian cartoonist living in Kitchener. He is best known for 'Cerebus', the groundbreaking comic book novel that recently concluded after a remarkable 300 issues.

Ruth Tait - pgs. 85 - 88

Rutz: (Ruth Tait) Rose many years ago out of the primeval ooze to become a vocational multi-tasking artist living and working in Toronto -- illustrator, animator, painter, storyboard artist, self and/or published comic book artist, teacher and writer. Look for her zines in all the best book stores in Toronto, that pander to such stuff. Website: www.artbyrt.com.

RG Taylor - pgs. 6 - 13, 52 - 56, 81 - 84, 89 - 92

Mississauga artist Richard G. Taylor was born in Fergus, Ontario.Richard taught elementary school for 27 years while enjoying a lively and productive career as an artist. His autobiographical cartoon strip, "The Blackboard Jumble" has appeared for 20 years in a variety of publications. He illustrated the critically acclaimed comicbook series "Wordsmith"and in the early nineties he drew "Sandman Mystery Theater" for D.C. Comics.

Quoc-Nghi Tran - pgs. 22 - 26
Born in Saigon, Viet-Nam in 1975, Quoc-Nghi, enrolled at Sheridan College in Ontario and participated in the Classical Animation Program in 1995. The following year he provided some work for DisneyTV Canada ("Beauty and the Beast: the Enchanted Christmas") and in 1997 was chosen to participate in a one month intensive Disney Boot Camp at CalState University in Monterey, California. After graduating at Sheridan College, he soon, he relocated from Toronto to Montreal and joined Cinar Animation Inc as a Layout Artist, Animator and Designer and worked briefly for Cine-Group Animation as a Storyboard Correction Artist. Quoc-Nghi continues to work at Cinar on children cartoons.

Noel Tuazon - pgs. - 72 - 73
A graduate of the Art and Art History at Erindale/Sheridan College but had better art education at a small animation school in downtown Toronto (Studio M). Comic book work has appeared in Arianne (2-issues), Taboo Especial, Dennis Eichorn's "Real Stuff", Frecklebean Comics and Art, and Reactor Girl. Has also illustrated for children's magazines Cricket, WeeOnes, and upcoming children's books produced by EECI, Inc.. Online portfolio can be viewed at:
www.portfolios.com/noeltuazon

Anthony Van Bruggen - pgs. 32 - 33
After a brief stint in comics in the mid-eighties, Anthony Van Bruggen spent fourteen years with the Walt Disney Company designing consumer products. He is currently VP of Creative for Thinkway Toys based in Markham, Ontario. A cancer survivor himself, Anthony is proud to contribute to this project. He dedicates his contribution to his wife, Caryn and their baby daughter, Hannah.

James Waley - pgs. 50 - 51
James Waley has been part of the Canadian comics scene for three decades. Beginning mid 70's as editor; art director; publisher and a writer/artist for ORB, a groundbreaking independent comic with early works by creators such as Gene Day, Ken Steacy and James Craig, he also showcased our first modern-era, non-satirical, national superhero, the Northern Light. The 80's saw Waley helming numerous productions for Heavy Metal; Charlton; Andromeda and Vortex, amongst others. A number of years managing comicons in Toronto and across Ontario he continued in comics with script and art direction on the Hudson's Bay Co.'s anniversary comic, TALES FROM THE BAY, and an ALI-BABA mini-series. Waley also created the FINE CANADIAN PANELLING column for ETC. magazine; articles for Parsec magazine and an online column for Internet Comics. He continues writing in, and about, comics along with helping to plan Paradise Comics' comicons and developing new comic productions. (jnw_pique@hotmail.com)

Rob Walton - pgs. 89 - 92
Rob Walton is a respected director and storyboard artist with over ten years experience in the animation industry. His comic books have been published to international acclaim including two Eisner Award nominations for his self-published work "Ragmop." Mr. Walton has written a screenplay based on his early series, "Bloodlines" which is currently being pursued as a feature film in Hollywood. Future plans include a return to comics and a live action short film to be shot in the summer of 2004.

Chip Zdarsky - pg. 49
Taking it to the max, while pushing it to the edge, Chip Zdarsky has extremely illustrated for an assortment of publications. He is currently hard at work on the next issue of Prison Funnies while completing his screenplay for Lord of the Rings 4.

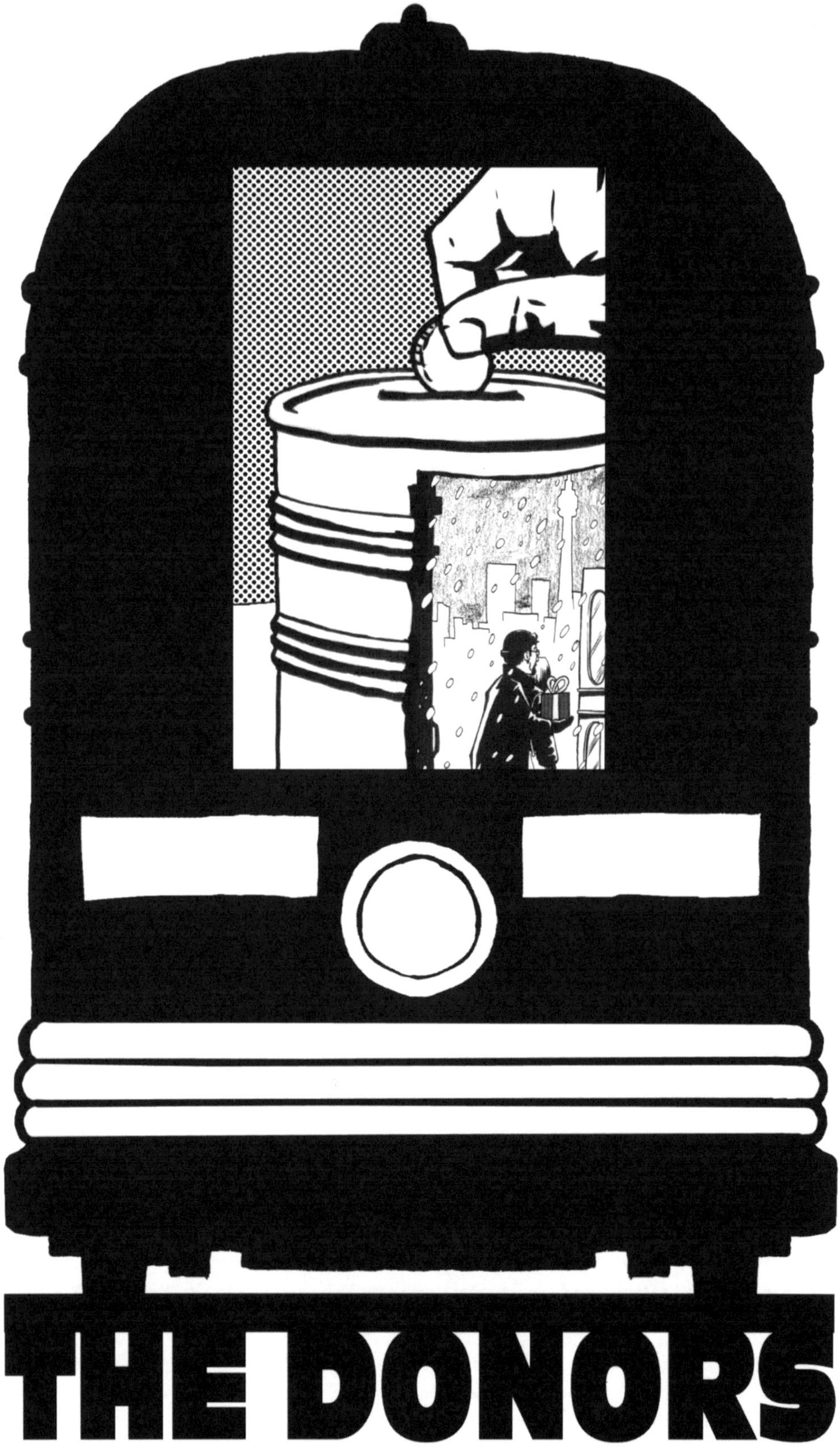

THE DONORS

This project was made possible by the private funding of the following donors. Without them, no one would be "Drawing The Line"; each person has made an immense difference.

Our deepest, heartfelt thanks and acknowledgment go to each of these extraordinary humanitarians...

Adam Brough

Allan Teichman

Alya & Sam Fattah

Andrew Lai

Angela & Jack Sheriton

Ann & Tony Eng

Ayda & Faruk Fattah

Barbara & Bill Farquhar

Barbara & Muwaffaq Fattah

Bessie & Jack Tang

Beth Baker

Bev & Jack Poulter

Blair Wynkoop

Börner-Jourdain Family

Boston-Bridger Family

Brian Morton

Bruce Peck

Candida Paltiel & Alex Moyle

Capital City Lodge #61, Knights of Pythias

Carol & Harry Steven Tang

Carol & Mark Gordon

Caroline & Khalid Fattah

Caroline Bamford & Patrick Watson

Cindy-Anne Eng & Paul Bendall

Claire & Paul Gratton

Daniel Stubbe

Davia Ezekiel

Dawn Michael & Kenneth Martin

Debbie & Ed Mar

Diane Bright

Donna & Daniel Zuckerbrot

Ducluzeau Family

Elizabeth & David Peck

Emily & Joseph Eng

Emmanuelle Gattuso & Allan Slaight

Erana & Ray Heard

Fely & David Kendall

Frances Colletti

Gabrielle & Jamie Hunter

Gad Caro

Galina Mohebat

Gwen & Keith Allison

Hera & Garo Kavoukian

Holly Arden & Doug Poruchny

Howard Alter

Ian Chamandy

Inci & Ihsan Cokgezer

Ingrid Reich & Bernie Michalik

Inoisell Miranda &
Michael Thiessen

Iryna Ivanova

Ish & Steve Lucas

Jan Howlett &
David Ben

Jane & Victor Eng

Jane & Willie Eng

Janice Cudlip &
Vladimir Torres

Jean & Gene Matsuura

Jean & George Chan

Joan & George Caesar

Julie Eng &
Suley Fattah

Karen Szulc &
Derek Snyder

Katinka Mastboom &
David Evans

Lara Fattah

Laura Dunn &
Robert Stofega

Laurent Comas

Laurie & Barrie Hayne

Linda & Eric Bedard

Lucy Guillet-Boyden &
Fred Boyden

Mac Hillier

Marina Duque &
Terence Queeley

Marion & Jack McBride

Mary Eng

Meredith Usher

Norma & Ed Silva-White

Pamela Kohly

Paola Saad

Parallel Production
Services Inc.

Pat Lyons

Phoebe Hancock &
Dan Morrissey

Phyllis & Herb Zarrow

Robin Kops

Roman Melichercik

Sabena Khan

Sabrina Chen-See

Sandra Eng

Sarrah Young

Selva Tuluy

Susie & Fenton Eng

Suus & Mark Mitton

Teresa Midbo &
Murray Hatfield

Trona Brady &
Dee Balkissoon

Valerie & Michael Adamo

Viktorya & Albert Tazbaz

Violet & George Golubov

Wynkoop-Tuluy Family

Zoe Isberg &
Jonathan Eng

Our sincere thanks and appreciation to the following companies for contributing to and supporting, Drawing The Line.

Aboveground Art Supplies
74 McCaul Street
Toronto, ON M5T 3K2
(416) 591-1601
www.abovegroundartsupplies.com

Central Reproductions Ltd.
4524 Eastgate Parkway
Mississauga, ON L4W 3W6
(905) 238-1250
www.central-repro.com

Frecklebean Café
126E McCaul Street
Toronto, ON
(416) 595-1943

Staples Business Depot (Store 25)
375 University Avenue
Toronto, ON M5G 2J5
(416) 598-4818
www.staples.ca

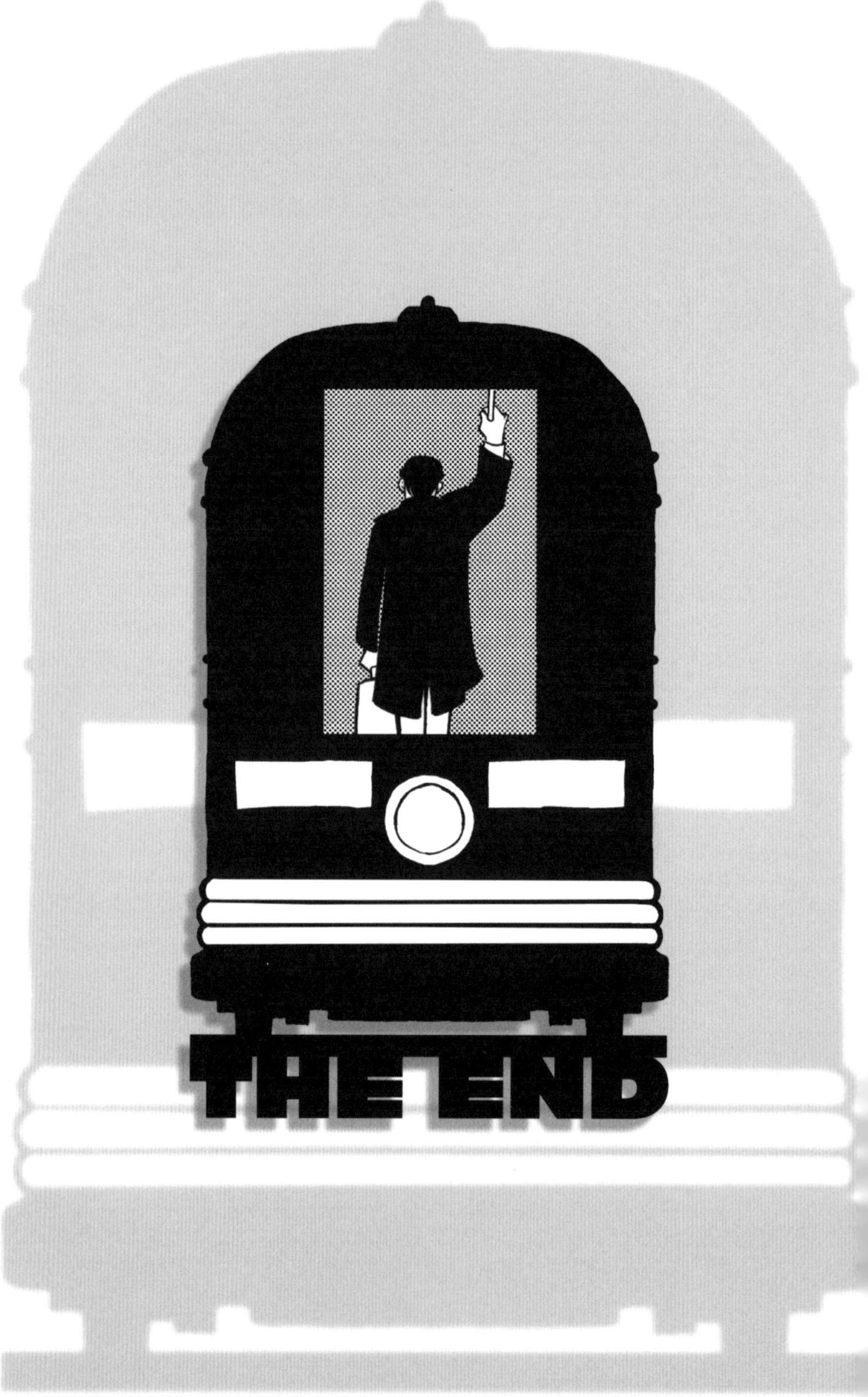
THE END

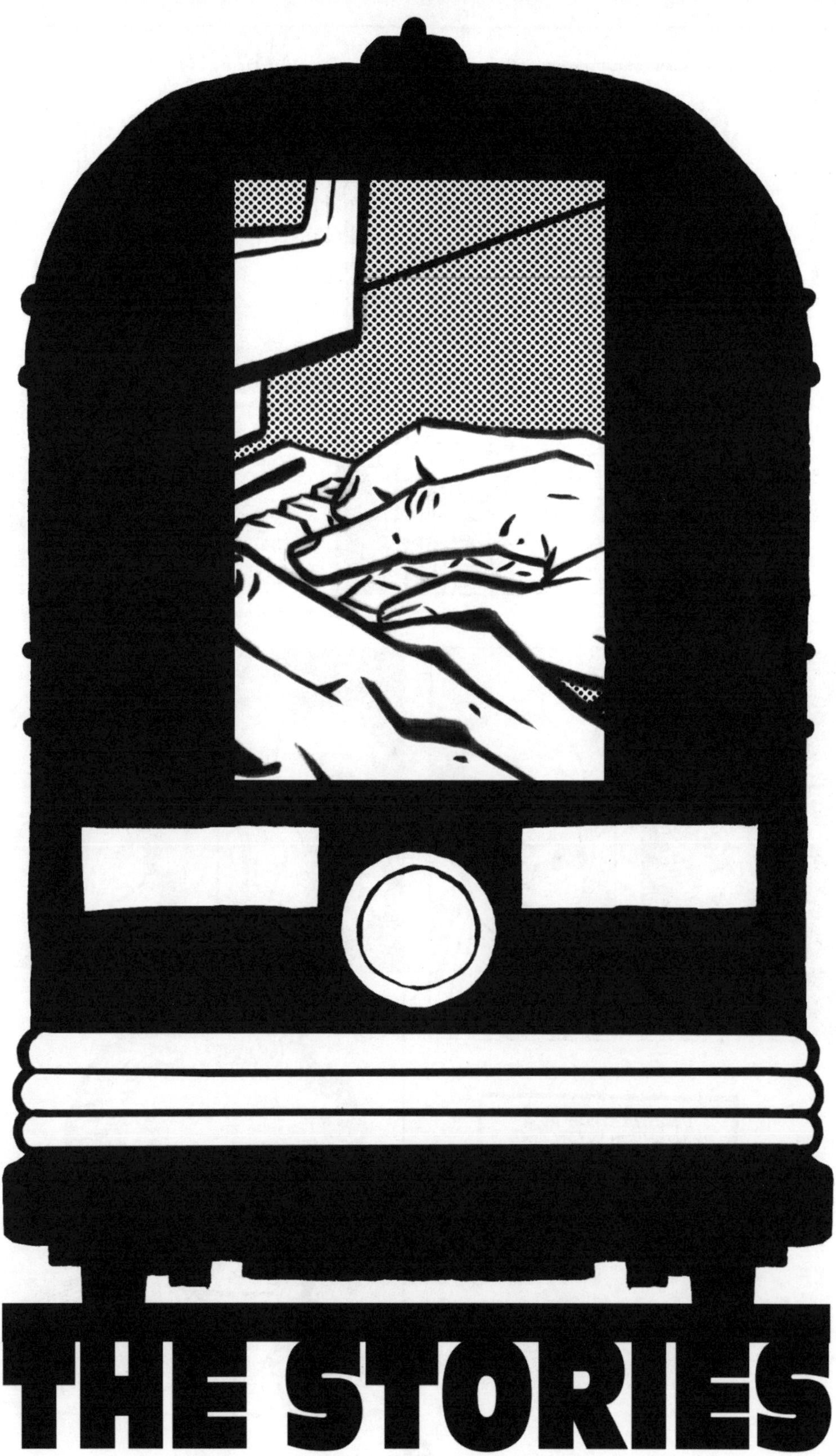

THE STORIES

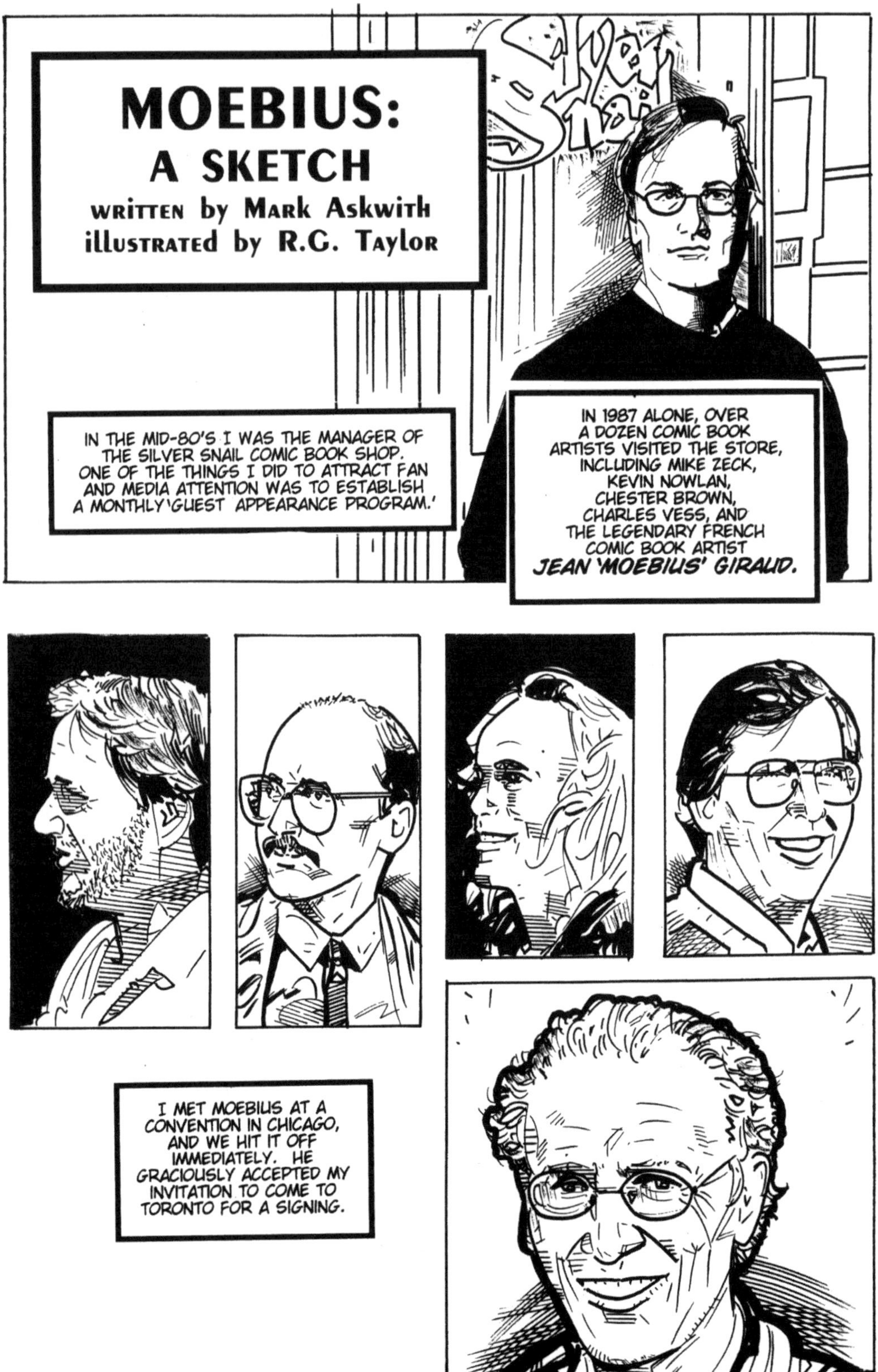
MOEBIUS:
A SKETCH
written by Mark Askwith
illustrated by R.G. Taylor
IN THE MID-80'S I WAS THE MANAGER OF THE SILVER SNAIL COMIC BOOK SHOP. ONE OF THE THINGS I DID TO ATTRACT FAN AND MEDIA ATTENTION WAS TO ESTABLISH A MONTHLY 'GUEST APPEARANCE PROGRAM.'
IN 1987 ALONE, OVER A DOZEN COMIC BOOK ARTISTS VISITED THE STORE, INCLUDING MIKE ZECK, KEVIN NOWLAN, CHESTER BROWN, CHARLES VESS, AND THE LEGENDARY FRENCH COMIC BOOK ARTIST JEAN 'MOEBIUS' GIRAUD.
I MET MOEBIUS AT A CONVENTION IN CHICAGO, AND WE HIT IT OFF IMMEDIATELY. HE GRACIOUSLY ACCEPTED MY INVITATION TO COME TO TORONTO FOR A SIGNING.

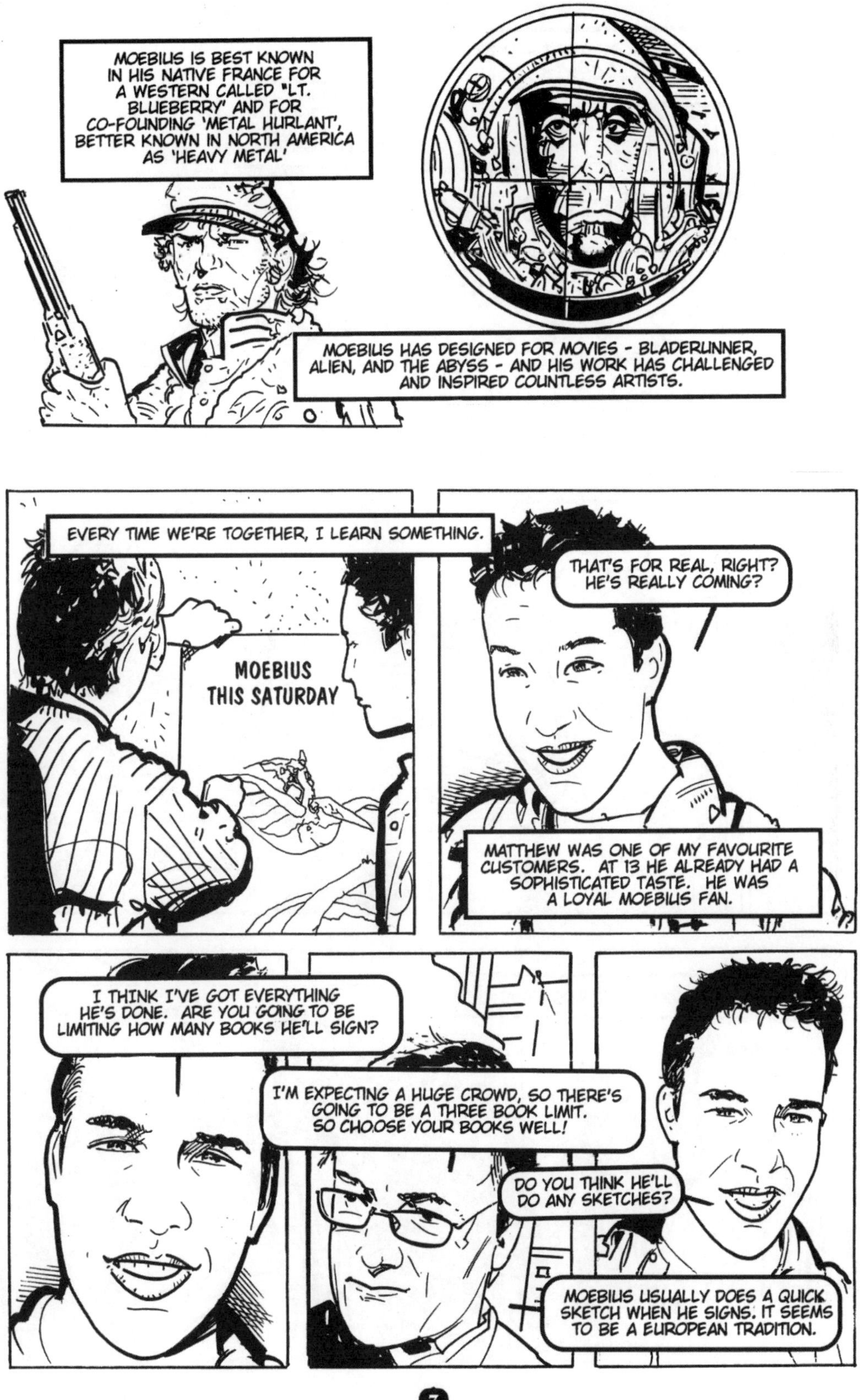
MOEBIUS IS BEST KNOWN IN HIS NATIVE FRANCE FOR A WESTERN CALLED 'LT. BLUEBERRY' AND FOR CO-FOUNDING 'METAL HURLANT', BETTER KNOWN IN NORTH AMERICA AS 'HEAVY METAL'
MOEBIUS HAS DESIGNED FOR MOVIES - BLADERUNNER, ALIEN, AND THE ABYSS - AND HIS WORK HAS CHALLENGED AND INSPIRED COUNTLESS ARTISTS.
EVERY TIME WE'RE TOGETHER, I LEARN SOMETHING.
MOEBIUS THIS SATURDAY
THAT'S FOR REAL, RIGHT? HE'S REALLY COMING?
MATTHEW WAS ONE OF MY FAVOURITE CUSTOMERS. AT 13 HE ALREADY HAD A SOPHISTICATED TASTE. HE WAS A LOYAL MOEBIUS FAN.
I THINK I'VE GOT EVERYTHING HE'S DONE. ARE YOU GOING TO BE LIMITING HOW MANY BOOKS HE'LL SIGN?
I'M EXPECTING A HUGE CROWD, SO THERE'S GOING TO BE A THREE BOOK LIMIT. SO CHOOSE YOUR BOOKS WELL!
DO YOU THINK HE'LL DO ANY SKETCHES?
MOEBIUS USUALLY DOES A QUICK SKETCH WHEN HE SIGNS. IT SEEMS TO BE A EUROPEAN TRADITION.

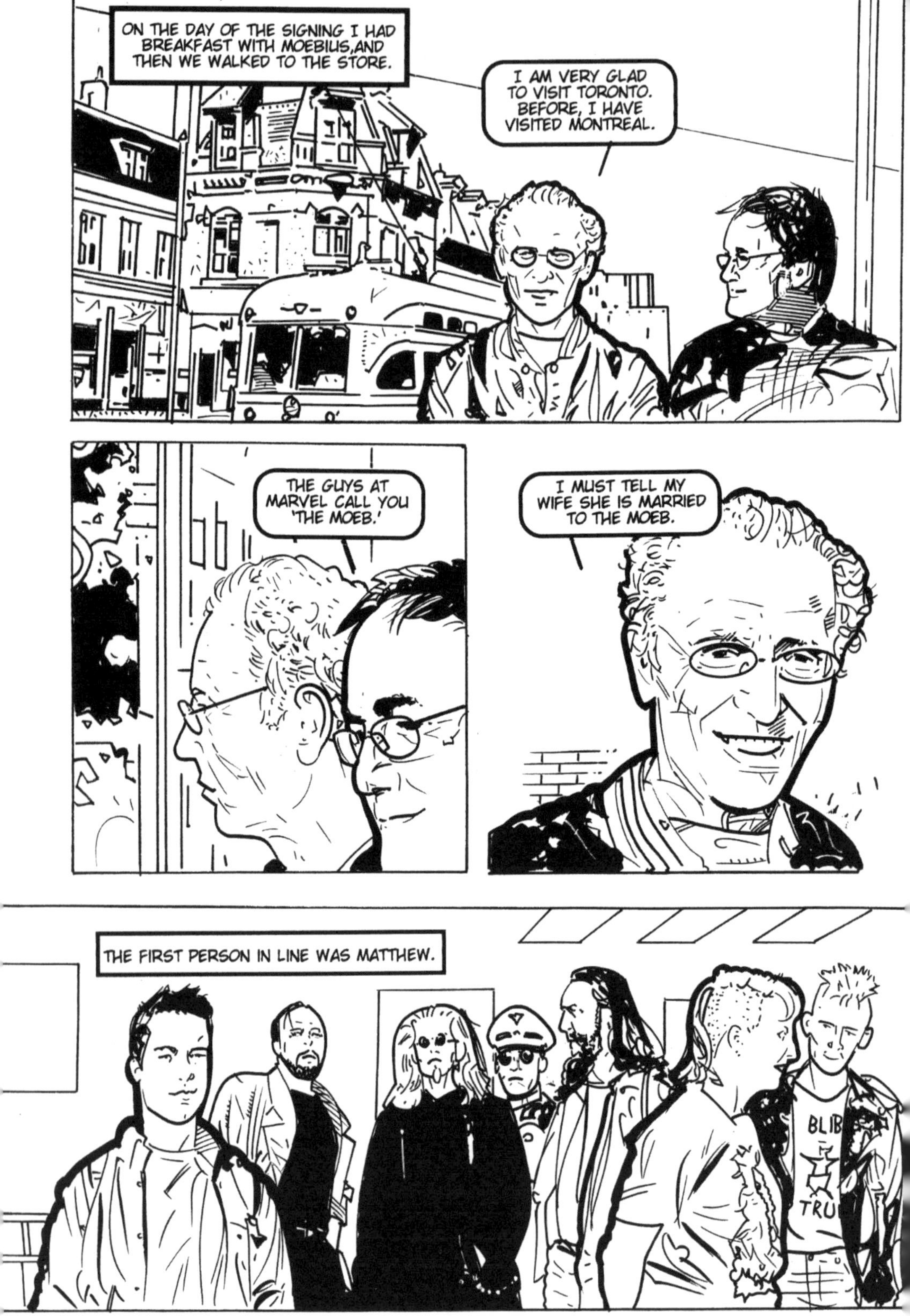
ON THE DAY OF THE SIGNING I HAD BREAKFAST WITH MOEBIUS,AND THEN WE WALKED TO THE STORE.
I AM VERY GLAD TO VISIT TORONTO. BEFORE, I HAVE VISITED MONTREAL.
THE GUYS AT MARVEL CALL YOU 'THE MOEB.'
I MUST TELL MY WIFE SHE IS MARRIED TO THE MOEB.
THE FIRST PERSON IN LINE WAS MATTHEW.

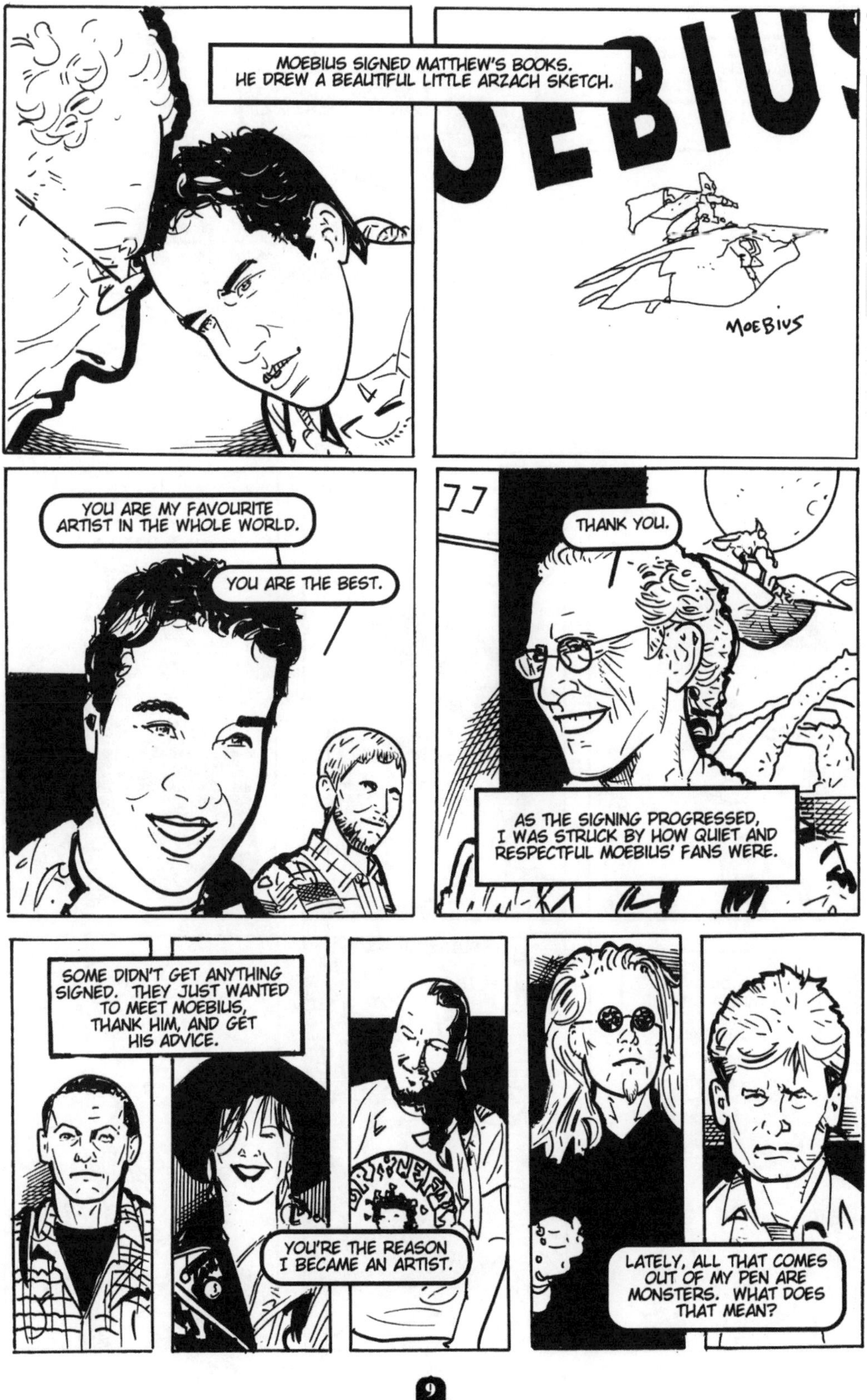
MOEBIUS SIGNED MATTHEW'S BOOKS.
HE DREW A BEAUTIFUL LITTLE ARZACH SKETCH.
OEBIUS
MOEBIUS
YOU ARE MY FAVOURITE ARTIST IN THE WHOLE WORLD.
YOU ARE THE BEST.
THANK YOU.
AS THE SIGNING PROGRESSED, I WAS STRUCK BY HOW QUIET AND RESPECTFUL MOEBIUS' FANS WERE.
SOME DIDN'T GET ANYTHING SIGNED. THEY JUST WANTED TO MEET MOEBIUS, THANK HIM, AND GET HIS ADVICE.
YOU'RE THE REASON I BECAME AN ARTIST.
LATELY, ALL THAT COMES OUT OF MY PEN ARE MONSTERS. WHAT DOES THAT MEAN?

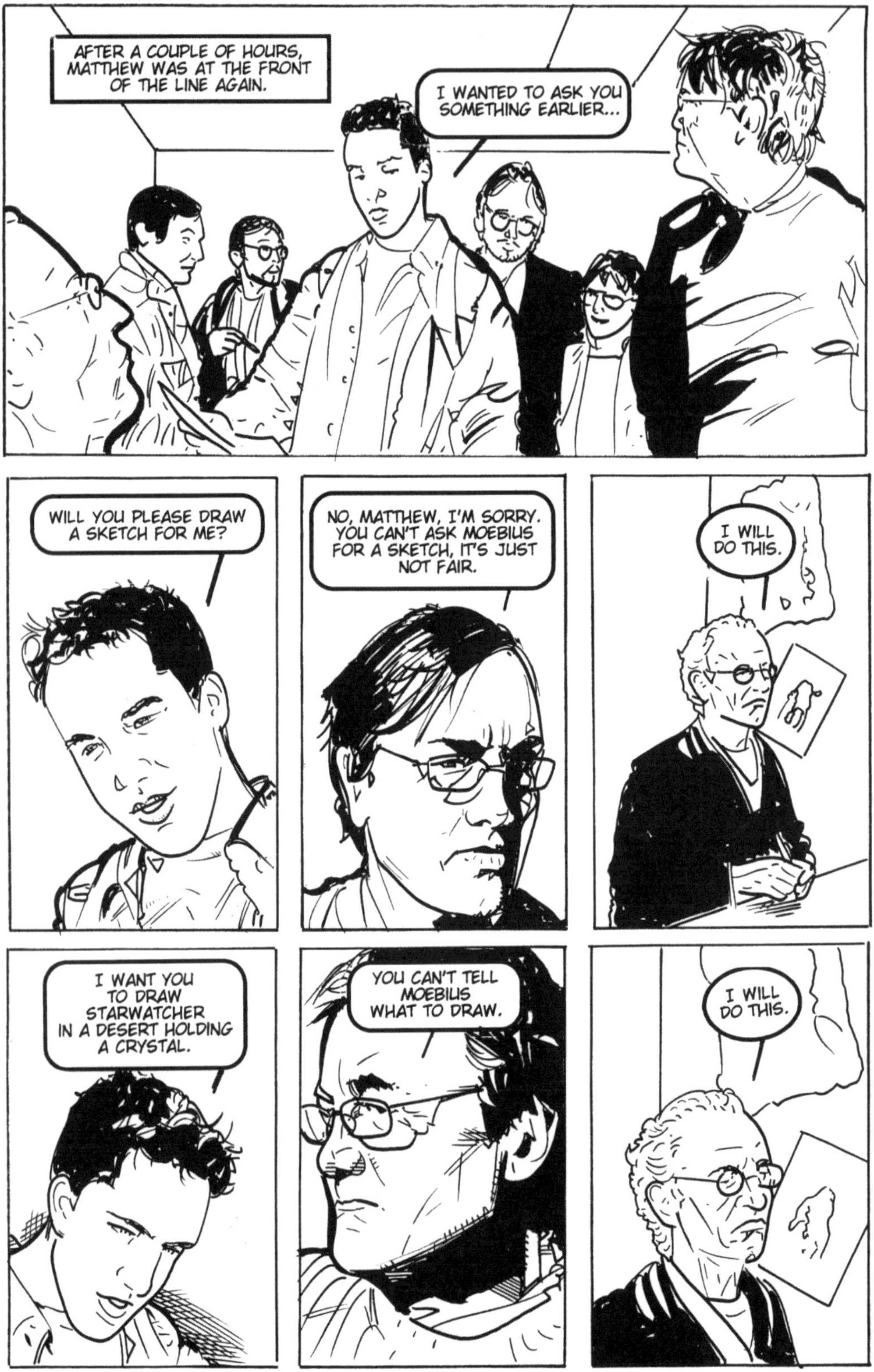
AFTER A COUPLE OF HOURS, MATTHEW WAS AT THE FRONT OF THE LINE AGAIN.
I WANTED TO ASK YOU SOMETHING EARLIER...
WILL YOU PLEASE DRAW A SKETCH FOR ME?
NO, MATTHEW, I'M SORRY. YOU CAN'T ASK MOEBIUS FOR A SKETCH, IT'S JUST NOT FAIR.
I WILL DO THIS.
I WANT YOU TO DRAW STARWATCHER IN A DESERT HOLDING A CRYSTAL.
YOU CAN'T TELL MOEBIUS WHAT TO DRAW.
I WILL DO THIS.

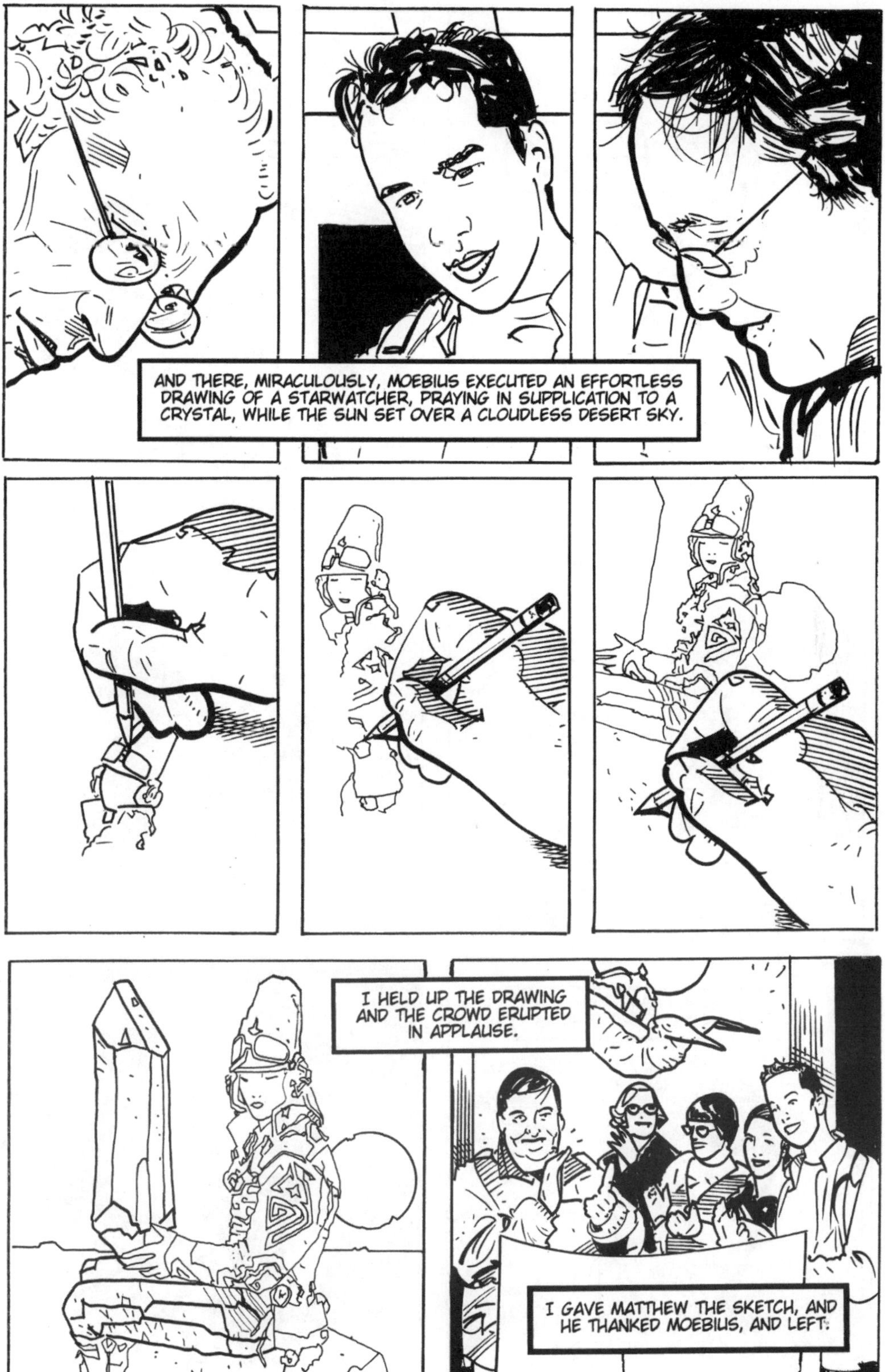
AND THERE, MIRACULOUSLY, MOEBIUS EXECUTED AN EFFORTLESS DRAWING OF A STARWATCHER, PRAYING IN SUPPLICATION TO A CRYSTAL, WHILE THE SUN SET OVER A CLOUDLESS DESERT SKY.
I HELD UP THE DRAWING AND THE CROWD ERUPTED IN APPLAUSE.
I GAVE MATTHEW THE SKETCH, AND HE THANKED MOEBIUS, AND LEFT.

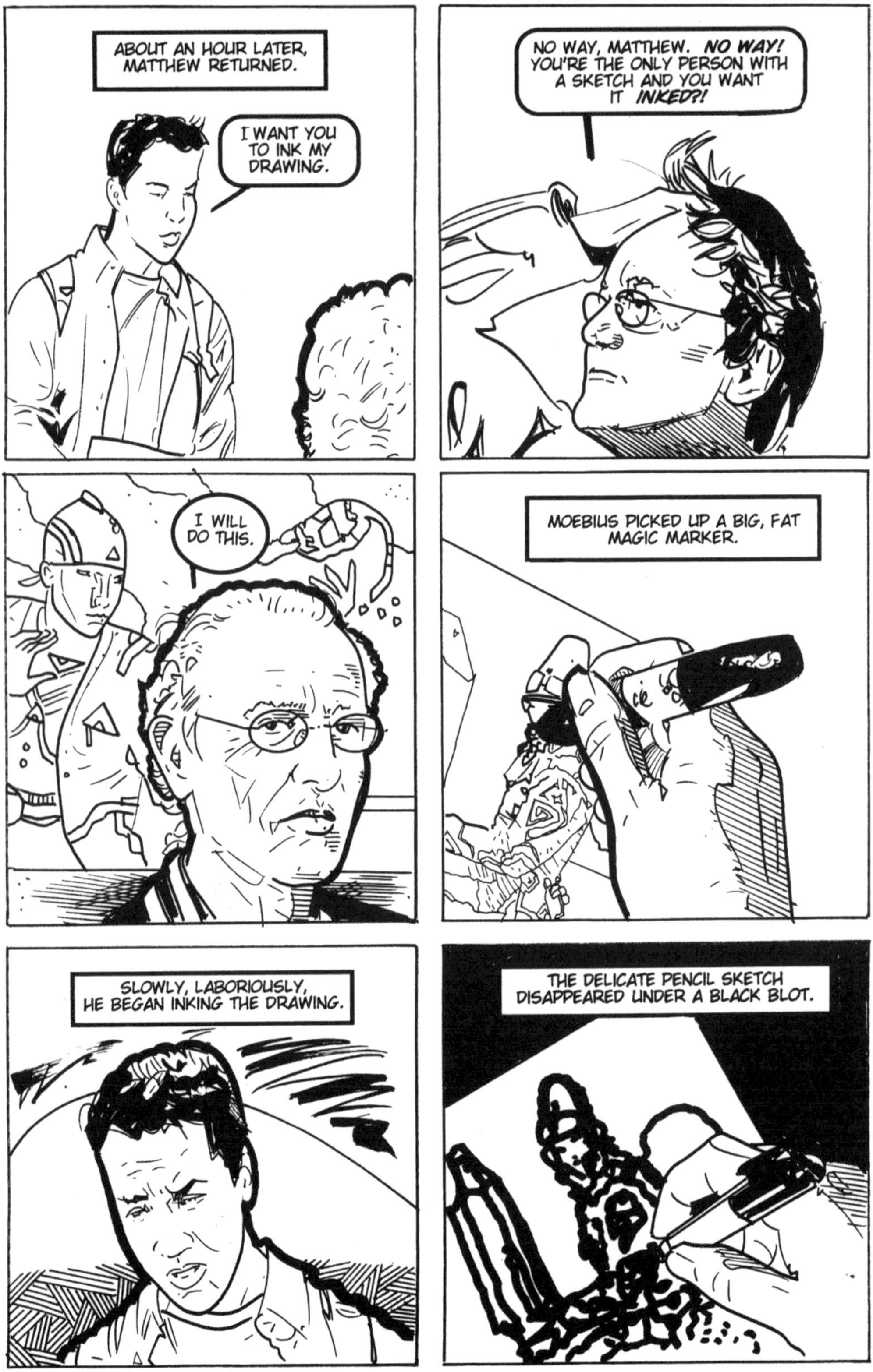
ABOUT AN HOUR LATER, MATTHEW RETURNED.
I WANT YOU TO INK MY DRAWING.
NO WAY, MATTHEW. NO WAY! YOU'RE THE ONLY PERSON WITH A SKETCH AND YOU WANT IT INKED?!
I WILL DO THIS.
MOEBIUS PICKED UP A BIG, FAT MAGIC MARKER.
SLOWLY, LABORIOUSLY, HE BEGAN INKING THE DRAWING.
THE DELICATE PENCIL SKETCH DISAPPEARED UNDER A BLACK BLOT.

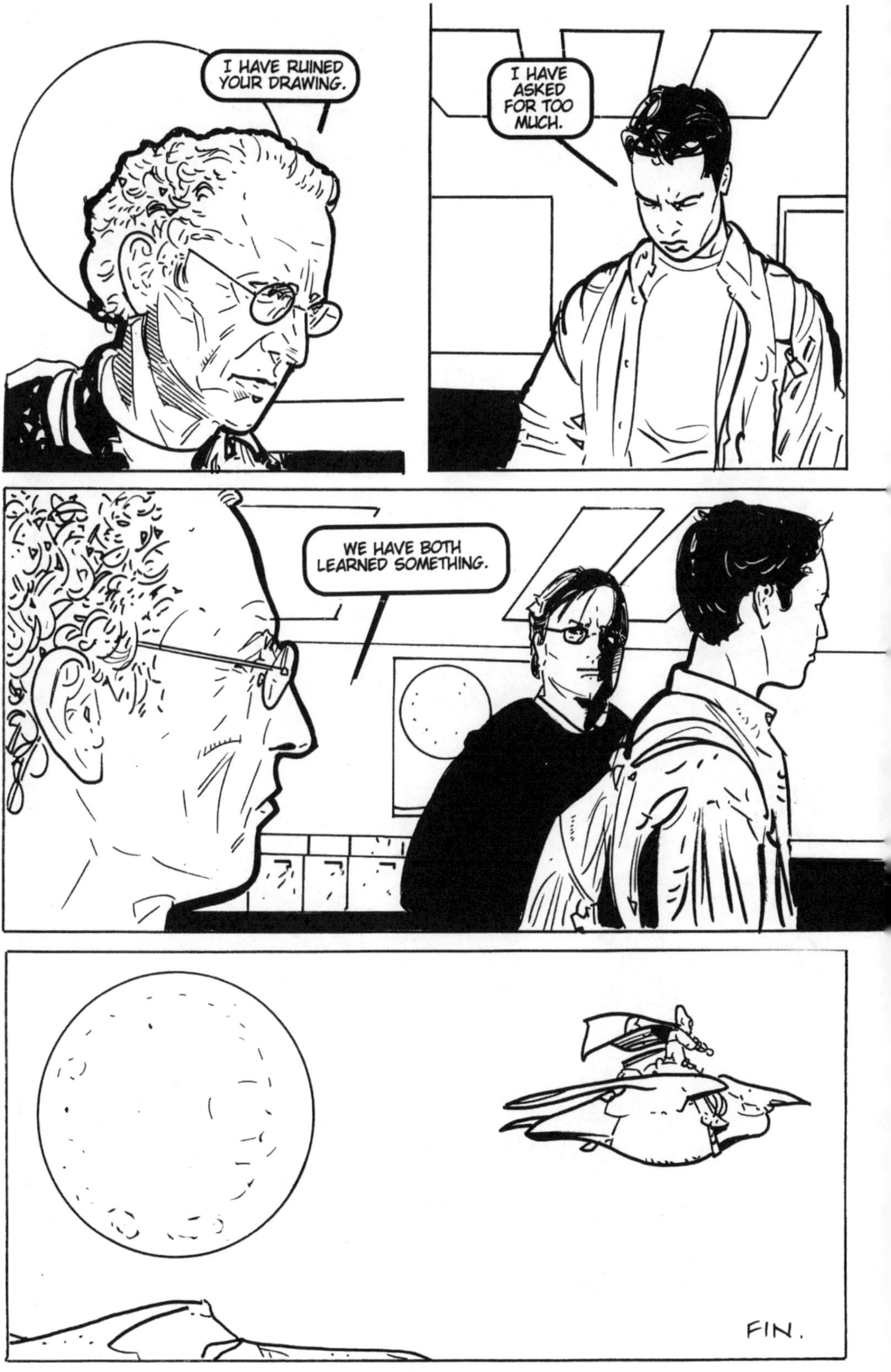
I HAVE RUINED YOUR DRAWING.
I HAVE ASKED FOR TOO MUCH.
WE HAVE BOTH LEARNED SOMETHING.
FIN.

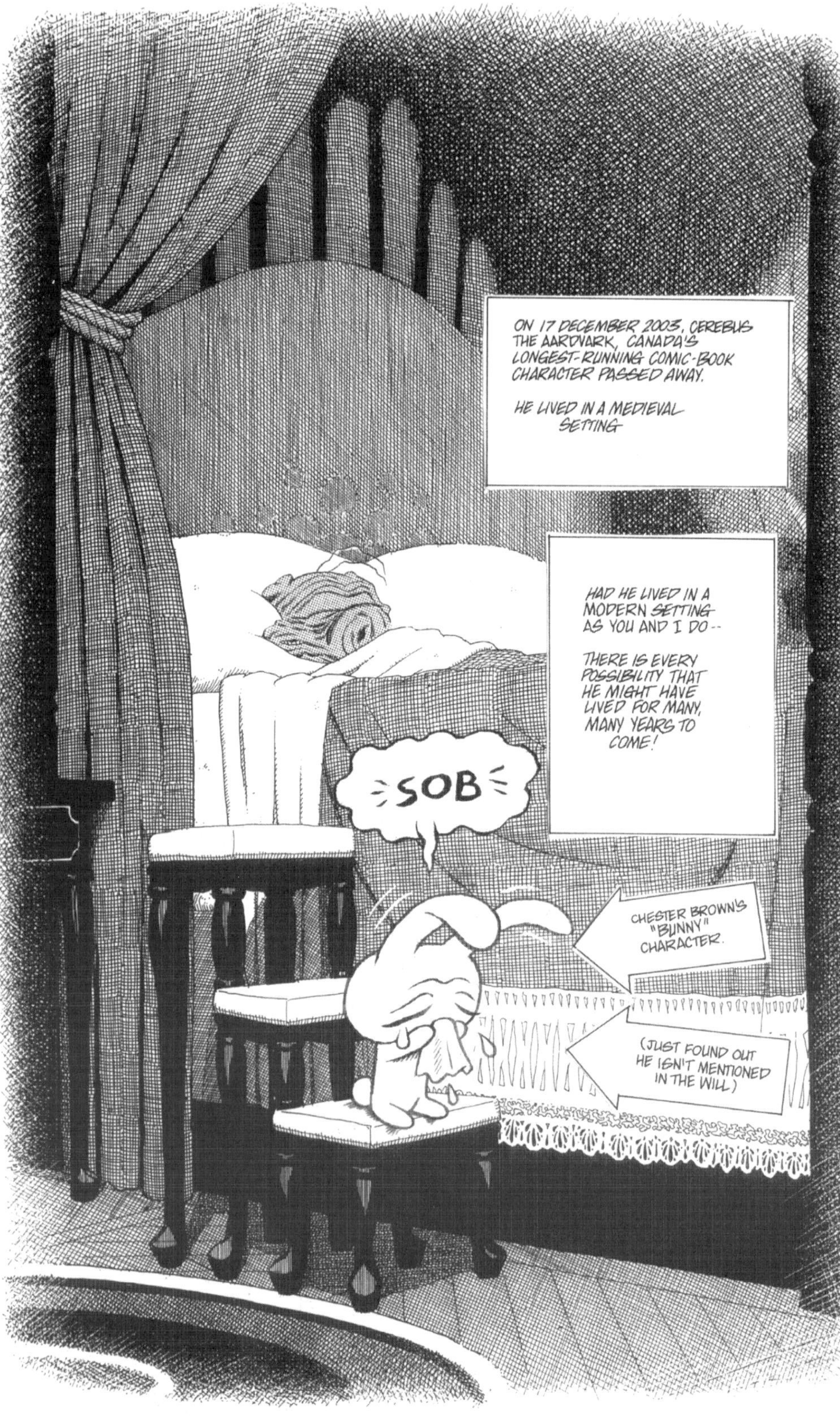
ON 17 DECEMBER 2003, CEREBUS THE AARDVARK, CANADA'S LONGEST-RUNNING COMIC-BOOK CHARACTER PASSED AWAY.
HE LIVED IN A MEDIEVAL SETTING
HAD HE LIVED IN A MODERN SETTING AS YOU AND I DO--
THERE IS EVERY POSSIBILITY THAT HE MIGHT HAVE LIVED FOR MANY, MANY YEARS TO COME!
SOB
CHESTER BROWN'S "BUNNY" CHARACTER.
(JUST FOUND OUT HE ISN'T MENTIONED IN THE WILL)

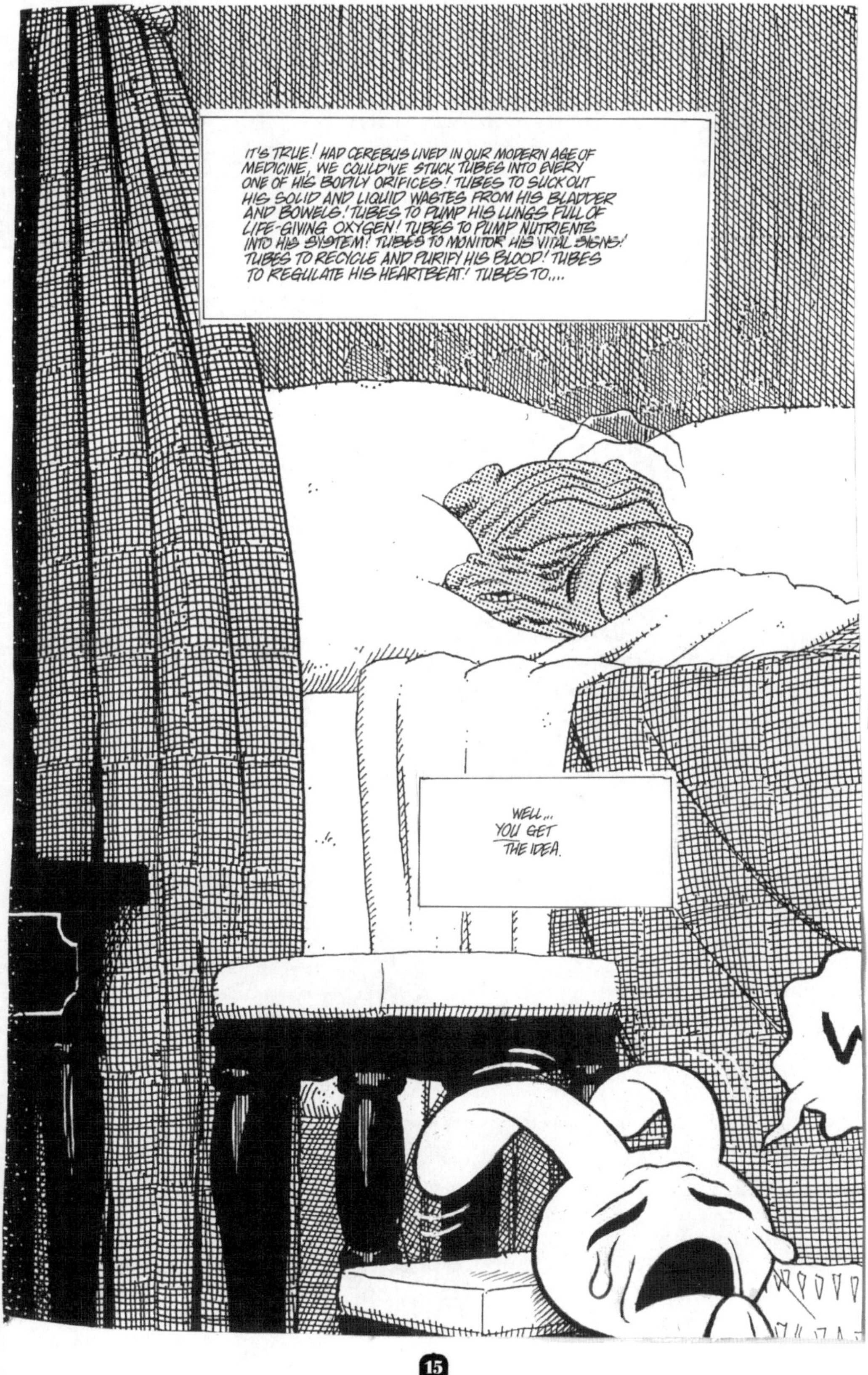
IT'S TRUE! HAD CEREBUS LIVED IN OUR MODERN AGE OF MEDICINE, WE COULD'VE STUCK TUBES INTO EVERY ONE OF HIS BODILY ORIFICES! TUBES TO SUCK OUT HIS SOLID AND LIQUID WASTES FROM HIS BLADDER AND BOWELS! TUBES TO PUMP HIS LUNGS FULL OF LIFE-GIVING OXYGEN! TUBES TO PUMP NUTRIENTS INTO HIS SYSTEM! TUBES TO MONITOR HIS VITAL SIGNS! TUBES TO RECYCLE AND PURIFY HIS BLOOD! TUBES TO REGULATE HIS HEARTBEAT! TUBES TO....
WELL... YOU GET THE IDEA.

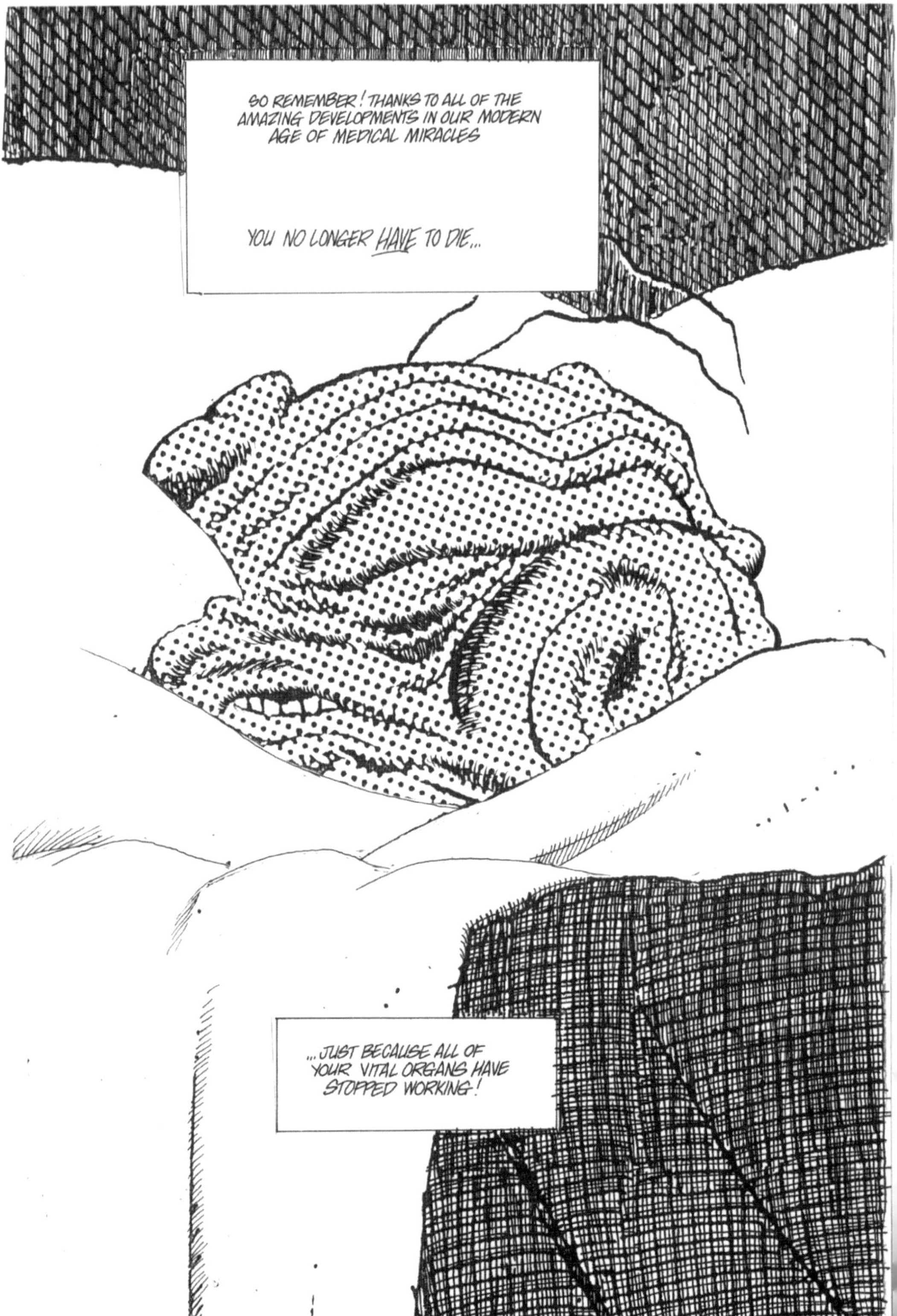
SO REMEMBER! THANKS TO ALL OF THE AMAZING DEVELOPMENTS IN OUR MODERN AGE OF MEDICAL MIRACLES
YOU NO LONGER HAVE TO DIE...
...JUST BECAUSE ALL OF YOUR VITAL ORGANS HAVE STOPPED WORKING!

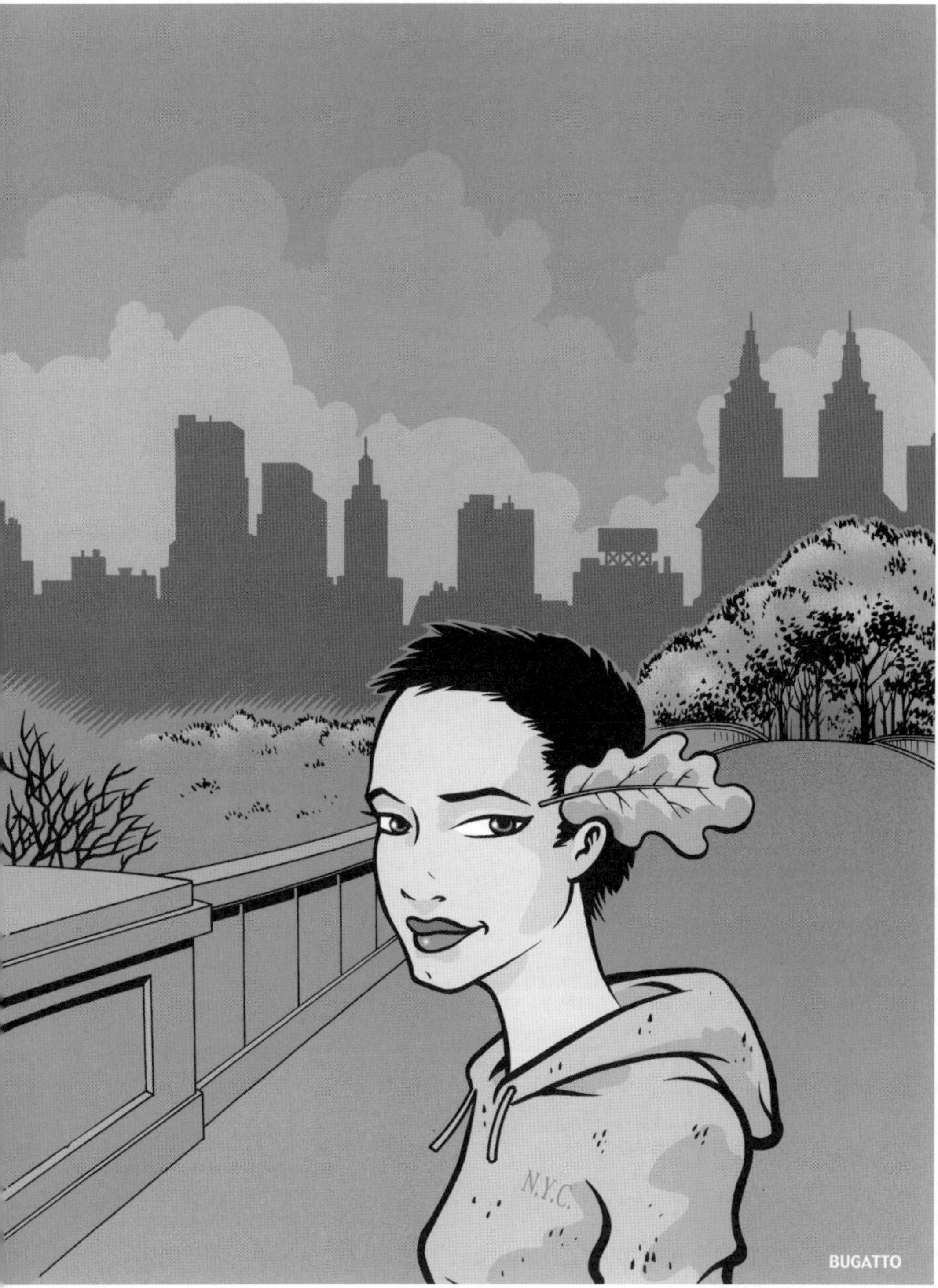
N.Y.C.
BUGATTO

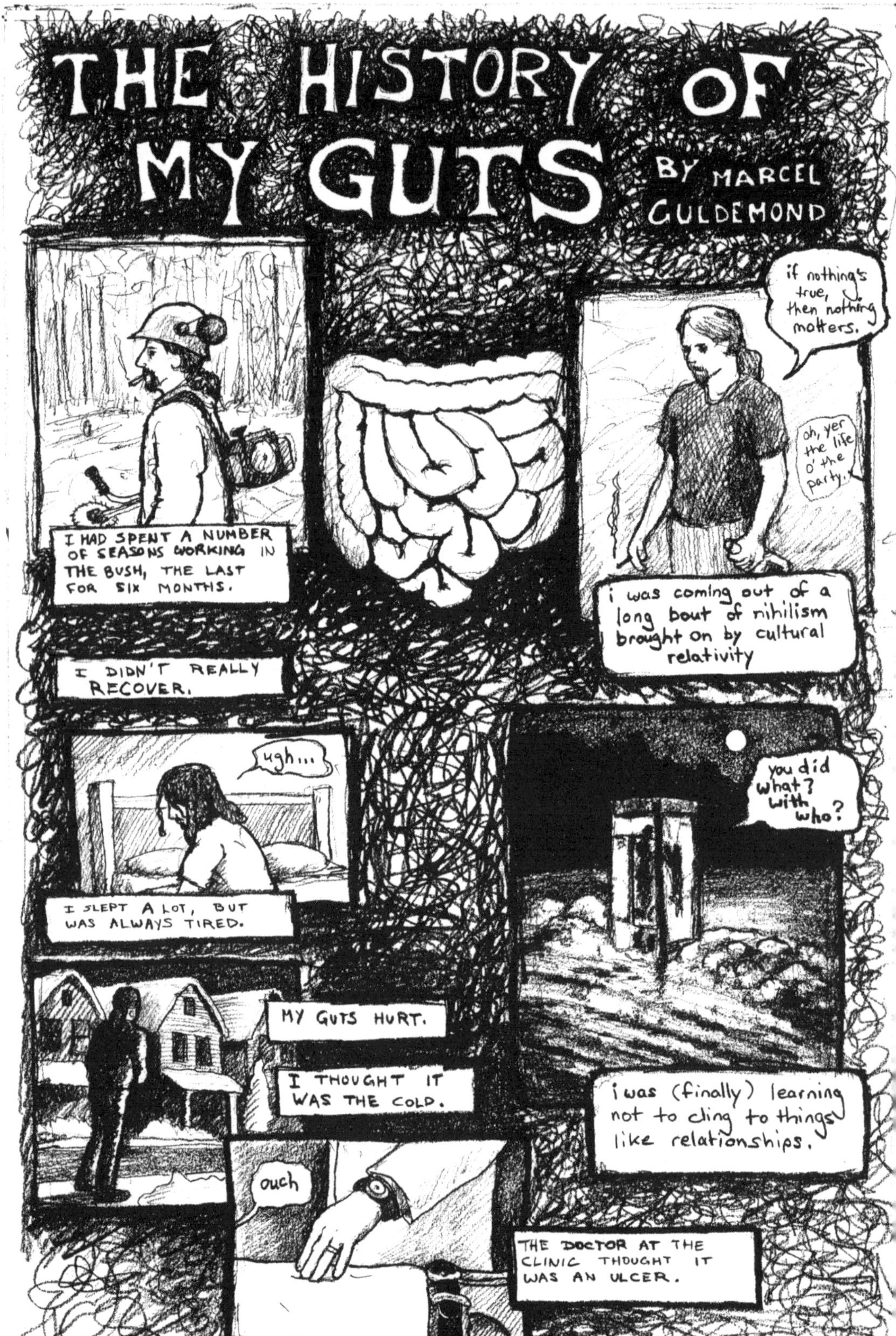
THE HISTORY OF MY GUTS
BY MARCEL GULDEMOND
I HAD SPENT A NUMBER OF SEASONS WORKING IN THE BUSH, THE LAST FOR SIX MONTHS.
I DIDN'T REALLY RECOVER.
if nothing's true, then nothing matters.
oh, yer the life o' the party.
i was coming out of a long bout of nihilism brought on by cultural relativity
ugh...
I SLEPT A LOT, BUT WAS ALWAYS TIRED.
you did what? with who?
MY GUTS HURT.
I THOUGHT IT WAS THE COLD.
i was (finally) learning not to cling to things like relationships.
ouch
THE DOCTOR AT THE CLINIC THOUGHT IT WAS AN ULCER.

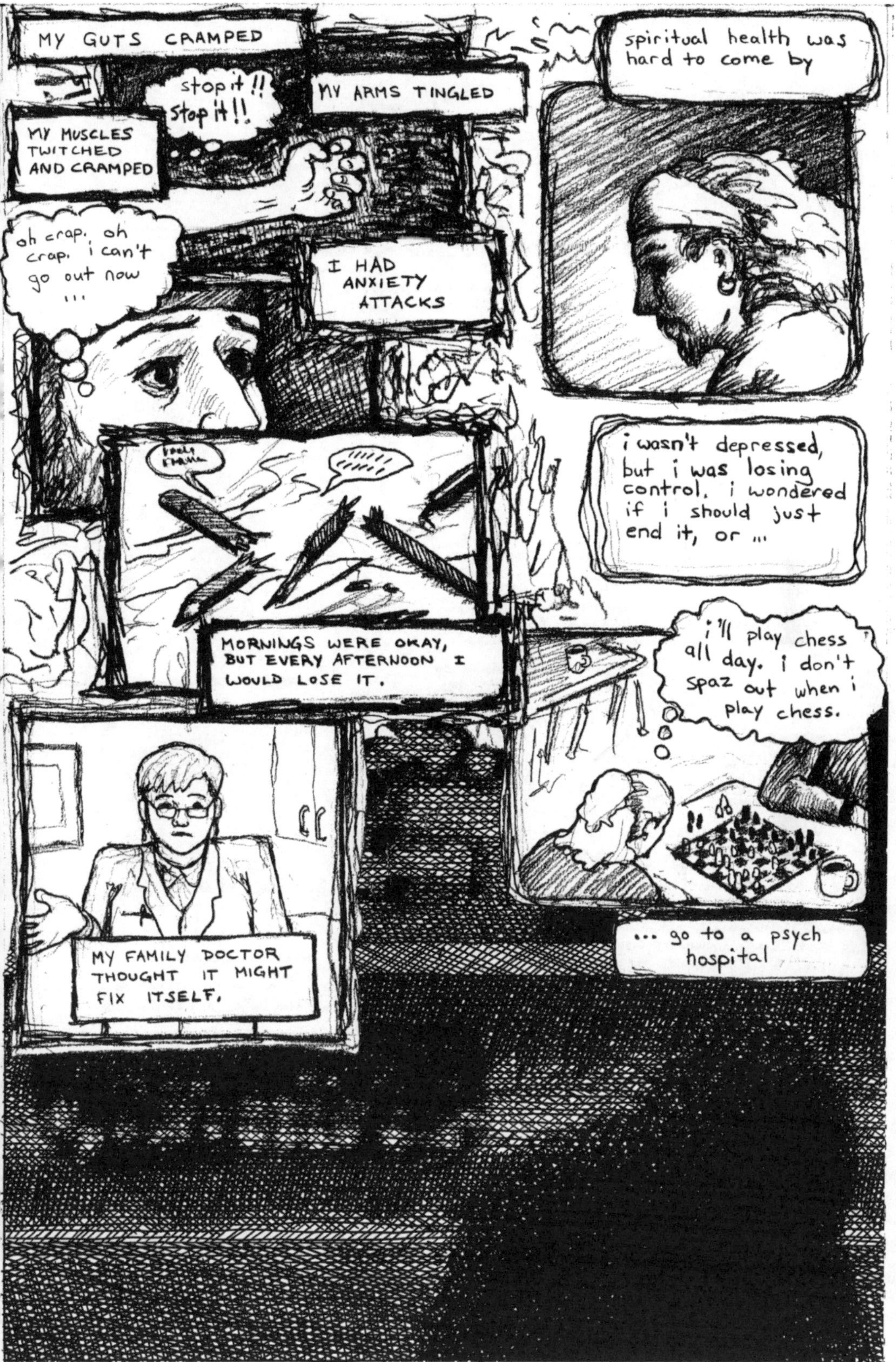
MY GUTS CRAMPED
stop it!! stop it!!
MY ARMS TINGLED
MY MUSCLES TWITCHED AND CRAMPED
oh crap. oh crap. i can't go out now ...
I HAD ANXIETY ATTACKS
MORNINGS WERE OKAY, BUT EVERY AFTERNOON I WOULD LOSE IT.
MY FAMILY DOCTOR THOUGHT IT MIGHT FIX ITSELF.
spiritual health was hard to come by
i wasn't depressed, but i was losing control. i wondered if i should just end it, or ...
i'll play chess all day. i don't spaz out when i play chess.
... go to a psych hospital

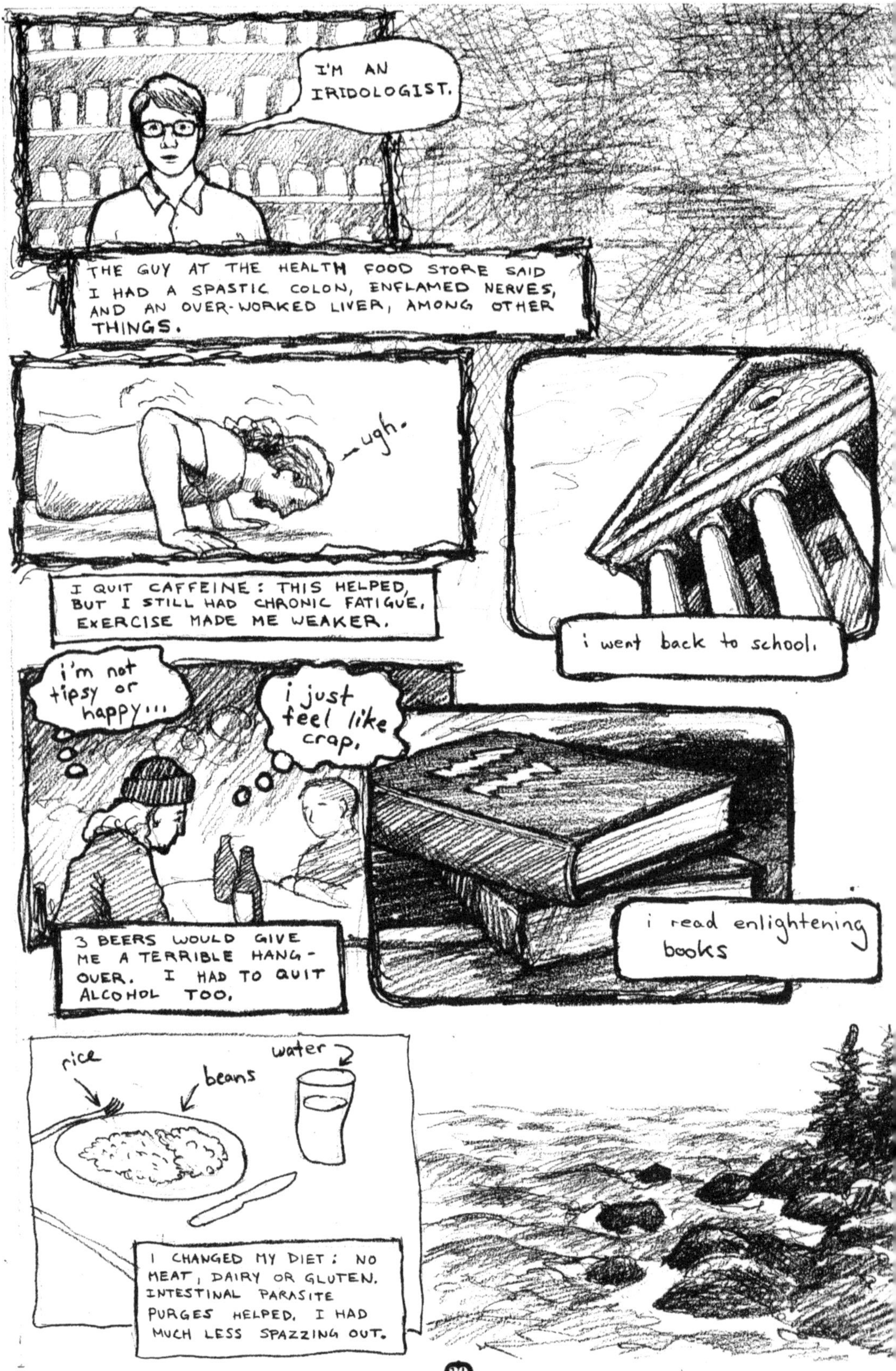

I'M AN IRIDOLOGIST.
THE GUY AT THE HEALTH FOOD STORE SAID I HAD A SPASTIC COLON, ENFLAMED NERVES, AND AN OVER-WORKED LIVER, AMONG OTHER THINGS.
ugh.
I QUIT CAFFEINE: THIS HELPED, BUT I STILL HAD CHRONIC FATIGUE. EXERCISE MADE ME WEAKER.
i went back to school.
i'm not tipsy or happy...
i just feel like crap.
3 BEERS WOULD GIVE ME A TERRIBLE HANG-OVER. I HAD TO QUIT ALCOHOL TOO.
i read enlightening books
rice
beans
water
I CHANGED MY DIET: NO MEAT, DAIRY OR GLUTEN. INTESTINAL PARASITE PURGES HELPED. I HAD MUCH LESS SPAZZING OUT.